Compassionate Mindful Inquiry
in Therapeutic Practice

of related interest

Practical Zen for Health, Wealth and Mindfulness
Julian Daizan Skinner with Sarah Bladen
Foreword by Shinzan Miyamae
ISBN 978 1 84819 390 1
eISBN 978 0 85701 347 7

The Compassionate Practitioner
How to Create a Successful and Rewarding Practice
Jane Wood
ISBN 978 1 84819 222 5
eISBN 978 0 85701 170 1

Words that Touch
How to Ask Questions Your Body Can Answer –
12 Essential 'Clean Questions' for Mind/Body Therapists
Nick Pole
ISBN 978 1 84819 336 9
eISBN 978 0 85701 292 0

The Four Qualities of Effective Physicians
Practical Ayurvedic Wisdom for Modern Physicians
Dr. Claudia Welch, DOM
Foreword by Dr. Robert Svoboda, BAMS
ISBN 978 1 84819 339 0
eISBN 978 0 85701 181 7

Getting Better at Getting People Better
Creating Successful Therapeutic Relationships
Noah Karrasch
ISBN 978 1 84819 239 3
eISBN 978 0 85701 186 2

COMPASSIONATE MINDFUL INQUIRY IN THERAPEUTIC PRACTICE

A Practical Guide for Mindfulness Teachers, Yoga Teachers and Allied Health Professionals

Karen Atkinson

Foreword by Vidyamala Burch

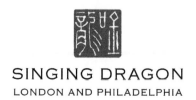

SINGING DRAGON
LONDON AND PHILADELPHIA

First published in 2020
by Singing Dragon
an imprint of Jessica Kingsley Publishers
73 Collier Street
London N1 9BE, UK
and
400 Market Street, Suite 400
Philadelphia, PA 19106, USA

www.singingdragon.com

Library of Congress Cataloging in Publication Data
A CIP catalog record for this book is available from the Library of Congress

British Library Cataloguing in Publication Data
A CIP catalogue record for this book is available from the British Library

ISBN 978 1 78775 175 0
eISBN 978 1 78775 176 7

Printed and bound in Great Britain

*To the Beacon Centre, for giving me
the opportunity to change my life.*

Contents

Foreword

Karen has written an important contribution to the evolving fields of mindfulness and compassion, both of which are seen as important methods to help alleviate suffering and enable people to live more rewarding lives.

All too often mindfulness and compassion are discussed as separate approaches in the belief that we can practice one or other of them in isolation. But, as Karen skilfully shows, it would be more accurate to describe them as two complementary and interrelated aspects of the lived experience of being whole, wise, kind and aware.

In some contemplative traditions, mindfulness and compassion are pictured as two wings of a bird. If a bird tries to fly with just one wing, it will surely never gain flight; we are the same. If we only practice mindfulness without its being imbued with kindness, we may end up with a dry, boring practice and soon give up. Compassion without awareness can easily become sentimentality or overwhelm. But compassionate mindfulness as a quality gives us the potential to become aware and kind, awake and connected. Surely these are beautiful qualities for any of us to aspire to.

Karen also generously shares her extensive experience with inquiry as a method for helping clients deepen their self-understanding and move towards growth and freedom. Inquiry is sometimes perceived as a mysterious, even intimidating, skill for the aspiring teacher to develop. Karen clearly and pragmatically de-mystifies it and introduces her Iceberg Model where awareness and compassion are allowed to unfold beautifully in the client through skilful and conscious 'open questioning' by the teacher, taking them through a series of distinct stages of growth.

Her colleague, Dr Trudi Edginton, has written Chapter 3 explaining the neuroscience behind our 'tricky brains'. She shows that our brains have evolved to be threat-based and that they are not particularly well adapted to the complexities of modern life. She goes on to demonstrate how compassionate mindfulness can profoundly change how our brains and nervous systems function. This enables us to respond to the inevitable stresses and difficulties of life in a more positive and healthy way. This chapter adds great richness to the book and Karen integrates it into her inquiry model, so it is clear which neurological functions are being activated at each stage.

It is obvious that Karen's approach to teaching and inquiry is based on many years of exploration and practice, as is her keen passion for teaching and helping people to make the most of their lives and experience. I am sure this book will be a great asset to the many professionals and teachers who wish to share these methods.

Vidyamala Burch

Acknowledgements

I am so very grateful to all those that have encouraged and supported me in writing this book. It has been 20 years of experience in the making, so I am unable to name all those who have contributed in so many ways. This includes all my clients, students, graduates, supervisors, supervisees and colleagues along the way. All your kindness and influence are appreciated and treasured.

Sincere appreciation to those from MindfulnessUK who have provided such huge support and encouragement, giving me the opportunity to take time away from the Centre and create the space to write. In particular, Angie Ward, who is a shining light in my life, Stephanie Unthank, who is uplifting and motivating, Anna Taylor, who makes my heart sing, and Kate Elliott, who kindly encourages me to play with the edge of my comfort.

A huge thank you to my talented son, Joel, of Gråskale Design, who did all the artwork and design, ensuring our thoughts and ideas came to life with his wonderful images.

Without my teachers guiding the way, helping me to change perspective, this book would not have been written. Thank you to Wendy Sullivan, Andy Wistreich, Shan Tate, Arabella Bowen, Geshe Tashi Tsering and Vanessa Hope.

To my friend, Dr Trudi Edginton of City University, London, you excited my brain with your neurological prowess, explaining my model with ease and clarity. Your expertise is phenomenal and I thank you from the bottom of my heart.

To Vidyamala, my admiration and fondness for you knows no bounds. I feel extremely honoured that you have written the Foreword for my book – thank you.

Thank you to the team at Jessica Kingsley Publishers. I have really appreciated your encouragement, your vision and your belief in me.

Finally, my husband, Neil, who has been my loving support and guide for over 30 years. I treasure you more than words can express.

Notes on the Text

Chapters 3 and 4 assume that the person reading the book is teaching mindfulness and compassion, and guiding inquiry.

Throughout the book I have referred to those being taught mindfulness and compassion as "clients". There is an understanding that they may also be known as "participants", "patients", "students" and other such terms.

The term "teacher" has been used in its broadest sense to incorporate therapists, healthcare workers, complementary medicine practitioners and anyone else who may be guiding inquiry within their own professional context.

The names of the clients and their specific circumstances have been changed to protect their anonymity, though the underlying "essence" is real.

I am not claiming that any of this material is new, but I have based this book on the model that I have developed, in the hope that inquiry will be seen as a crucial teaching skill that can be honed and developed over time. The Iceberg Model sets out to explain the relationship between mindfulness and compassion in a practical and sequential way, allowing for the growth and development of both the teacher and the client as they walk side by side through this process.

Chapter 1

EXPLORING COMPASSIONATE MINDFUL INQUIRY

Inquiry lies at the heart of our work as mindfulness teachers. However, it is not mindfulness alone that serves us here. Inquiry is the place in which we receive the experiences of our students, offering both a grounded and caring presence that encourages them to explore difficulty gently, beginning to let go of previously held beliefs about themselves and their lives. We enter alongside them into this new and often shaky place of not-knowing, keeping our hearts open, not pulling away but allowing whatever is present. It is this mindful and compassionate holding by the teacher that offers students the possibility that even great challenges can be met in this way in their own lives.

Vanessa Hope[1]

The potential for healing and change promised by inquiry excites, and the outcomes constantly astound me. The reason I love this part of teaching is because it is such a privilege to help facilitate and observe acceptance and subsequent change from the gentle, soft beginnings in this most tender-hearted work: the unveiling of vulnerabilities, working with places of resistance, barriers and edges, to explore what is really going on. This enhances lives in so many subtle ways and, for some, it can be totally life-changing, as it was for me. Slowly, slowly,

---

1   Personal communication (2019) with Vanessa Hope (mindfulness and mindful self-compassion teacher and trainer).

the time spent practising and inquiring can open up a whole new freeing world of choices, love and connectivity.

Sometimes the teacher needs to go gently, but sometimes the questions can be edgy, challenging, nudging a client on whilst holding the compassionate space, in order to explore and gain a wider perspective and enable the opportunity to see things as they really are. Inquiry supports people in their lives in extraordinary ways, facilitated by a compassionate, mindful inquirer.

Inquiry manifests itself as different things, in some respects, at different times. I adjust my skills around inquiry according to the client, where they are with their understanding of themselves, their learning, their ability to be insightful and what's happening for them in their lives at that particular point in time. And that's the key: inquiry is not going back over old ground, ruminating and re-igniting difficulties or old wounds; nor is it projecting into the future, trying to make something happen in a goal-orientated way. Compassionate mindful inquiry explores what is happening right now, in this moment, on any level, be it superficial or at the depths of one's being. This is the absolute, pure joy. It can be guided with anyone, at any age, with or without experience, after any practice.

As this book sets out to show, there's not just one, formulaic way of guiding inquiry and there's absolutely no right or wrong way to lead it. So long as the inquirer has an open heart, is humble and fully present with the other person, in a natural, authentic way, then the client will have the opportunity to explore, to a greater or lesser extent, what their experiences were during their practice.

Nor is there a specific setting that is of more benefit than another. Throughout my career, mindfulness and compassion have underpinned all my work, ranging from nurse to yoga teacher, complementary practitioner, therapist, teacher and teacher trainer. The beauty of these approaches is that they complement every field of work equally and can be taught in such a vast range of ways to support not only our fellow humans but also the animals we care for, the food we grow and the environment in which we live, through the choices we make and the nurture we bring to these interdependent relationships.

What is important is that the teacher does not need to take on the responsibility of needing to fix things or make them different from how they already are. Change often occurs indirectly in response to observing and holding what is already present, with kindness and compassion.

Having said this, the experience of the teacher informs the level of inquiry and their ability to guide it skilfully, exploring, unfolding, discovering and facilitating change, growth and freedom in innumerable ways. The process is never boring as the teacher never knows what the client is going to say or what the outcome from the process will be. It's an unending delight to facilitate and guide others in this way: listening to the beauty of their descriptions about their experiences, and witnessing their courage to explore deeper into the unknown and the ramifications of what is discovered in order to develop the resources to support themselves fully and with kindness.

In the busyness of the world in which we live it can often feel like there is no time to sit and contemplate. Practice has such a special, unique quality, and inquiry enables that quality to be revealed and articulated in a way that just thinking about things cannot touch.

The whole process of practice, plus inquiry, plus incorporating what is revealed and learnt into life, has endless possibilities, which is what makes it so exciting and deserving of appreciation, care and consideration. Developing inquiry after practising mindfulness is what creates long-lasting and profound change; it is such a powerful and undervalued teaching tool and as such requires targeted attention during the teacher training process and beyond, when teaching to others. I see inquiry as assisting clients in the identification of resources they already have, as well as in the development of new ones. For some, inquiry can be like the icing on the cake, enriching existing resources more fully; for others, inquiry creates the building blocks which make them stronger, provide the foundation to shore them up in times of difficulty, and enable them to flourish.

Awareness is a one-way street, so once these new, insightful ways of perceiving events, dealing with difficulties or behaving contrary to habitual patterns are discovered, explored, validated and learnt, they cannot be unlearnt. This incentivises clients, giving them the courage to continue discovering new ways of living life and creating fresh and new ways of being.

A spontaneous and non-cognitive response during inquiry comes from deep within and is certainly where the juice is. I often sense myself responding in a guttural way when this event is happening, resonating with what is being said and holding the space delicately for whatever might arise for the client. This is a precious moment, something to be savoured, a place of authentic learning and growth.

One of my supervisees, James Murray,[2] has just told me:

> Inquiry is everything. It's not actually the words they feed back after experiencing a practice that's important, but the root, the origin of these words. Facilitating the recognition and understanding of this root can lead to a gentle yet profound change in the participant's experience of themselves, culminating in developing the capacity to make more effective and supportive choices in the way they live their lives.

The *Collins English Dictionary* (2019) describes inquiry as "a question which you may ask in order to get some information". This is it, in essence, but inquiry explores more deeply and specifically into the nature of the mind and the effects this has on the body and emotions, leading us to think, feel and act in the way that we do.

This capacity to be able to facilitate clients seeing the truth or reality of the situation, letting go of the stories, patterns and resistance to change, as well as the teacher's role in not trying to fix things, make things better or provide a solution, is what makes this teaching unlike any other role. It comes as a great relief to trainees and new teachers to appreciate that they don't need to have all the answers and that, although mindfulness is therapeutic in nature, it's not a therapy, so they can let go of the requirement to "get it right".

I do hope that it is becoming very apparent that leading inquiry is more than just a conversation between two people. It is the employment of a vast range of skills with the aim of deepening understanding as well as providing tools to work with whatever arises.

Jon Kabat-Zinn and Saki Santorelli (1999, p.16) explain that "this requires the instructor to sharpen his/her ability to listen closely, allow space, refrain from the impulse to give advice, and instead, to inquire directly into the actuality of the participants' experience".

The word "inquiry" may seem a little harsh, invasive and confrontational, but prefixing it with the words "compassionate" and "mindful" softens it and adds context to the whole process. Up to a point, this is about semantics, but I do think the attitude that the teacher brings

---

2   Personal communication (2019) with James Murray (mindfulness teacher).

to the process changes the tone so that inquiry becomes more of a process, whereby the teacher is walking alongside the client rather than taking a position of being an expert or assuming a position of authority.

McCown, Micozzi and Reibel (2011, p.127) describe this interaction, saying "Much of the transformative effects of the MBIs [Mindfulness-Based Interventions] may be potentiated by dialogue encounters with participants".

The process is guided with curiosity and humility. Interestingly the words "curiosity" and "humility" are derived from the Latin words *cura* (care) and *humus* (ground or earth), respectively. If the teacher is curious and humble, they are earthed and grounded when guiding inquiry with a caring attitude.

One of the most important things a teacher must do to develop these qualities is have their own regular mindfulness practice. This is what is drawn upon to begin the process of inquiry, embodying mindfulness, exhibiting a non-judgemental, curious and attentive presence with kindness.

Gary Heads, author of *Living Mindfully* (Heads 2017) and a personal friend of mine, talks of how an individual must spend hours and hours of work on a piano, and investigate their instrument over many, many years in order to become a jazz pianist who improvises in the moment according to mood, venue and audience. This is truly how it is to conduct the process of inquiry: the more practice and effort put into honing inquiry skills, the more the teacher is able to improvise and conduct it with skill and competence to elicit sustainable, transformative changes.

Mindfulness

The term "compassionate mindful inquiry" refers to the skilful facilitation of inquiry by a teacher after a mindfulness practice, and the exploration of the effects of compassion and kindness in the whole process.

Mindfulness is a practice which involves choosing an object on which to rest attention. This sounds so simple, but minds, as we know, have a tendency to wander; so when practising, one recognises the wandering mind and brings attention back to the object over and over again, with attitudes of curiosity and kindness. This chosen object may be the breath, the body, sounds, a colourful crystal, thoughts, emotions or whatever it is that arises in the field of awareness in the present moment.

Through building the capacity to come back to the chosen object time and again, whilst creating an awareness of thoughts, physical sensations and emotions in the body during the practice, the individual develops a deeper understanding regarding tendencies, habits of mind and subsequent behaviour, thereby gaining perspective and clarity. This then creates an opportunity for change and transformation. Mindful awareness and the building of the capacity to return time and again to the object are integral to the process and a key starting point for all.

Some people teach mindfulness simply as bare attention, but there is more to it than this. Awareness and attention control strengthen the mental muscle and help us to become more connected to ourselves. A phrase I often use is "We're grown-ups now and we have a choice to continue to live our lives as determined by the habits we developed as children or to become adults and take some responsibility for how we think, feel and behave." As such, we have the capacity to sense into[3] the freedom of spaciousness by moving away from the learnt and embedded patterns, peeling away the layers of defence and resistance to see things with fresh eyes and realise our full potential.

Noticing the external distractions and our propensity to become attached to these stimuli can be identified through practice, as attention is consciously transferred inwards from gross consciousness (involved during chatting, planning and doing) to the more subtle and nuanced aspects of consciousness, sometimes tapping into the subconscious to unveil what truly informs and drives us. Seeing this clearly provides the springboard from which to change and consequently increases our levels of joy and happiness.

Compassion
The words "compassion" and "self-compassion" can conjure up all sorts of images and feelings of guilt, selfishness, navel-gazing and

---

3   Using all the senses, including the "felt sense" and emotions, to connect with the experience more fully. The emphasis is taken away from thinking and is instead focused on feeling, which minimises judgement and criticism and helps to connect with what is really here, right now.

even narcissism. They can also be associated with the term "compassion fatigue", which presupposes that we have finite amounts of compassion and that using this up leads to ill-health and collapse. As I sit back and consider this Western view, I only have to think of people such as the Dalai Lama and Mother Teresa to see that this concept is inaccurate, as their compassion for others seems cumulative and boundless.

If you think about it, making a conscious choice to do a mindfulness practice is, in itself, an act of self-compassion. So, you see, mindfulness and compassion are inextricably linked. One cannot be separated from the other, even though in this secular, medicalised, evidence-based world in which we live, mindfulness is heralded as something quite different and sometimes entirely disconnected from compassion.

Their connection lies in viewing mindfulness as more about the observation of an experience, whereas compassion shifts attention more towards the experience itself and how the client engaged with the experience.

A compassionate mindfulness practice sets the intention of bringing a soft and kindly attitude to whatever arises during, or in response to, practice. If judgement (for example, in the form of self-criticism) arises, bringing some self-soothing phrases into the practice or self-inquiry can have a profoundly beneficial effect. It may be that the client begins to observe that there is a distinct lack of self-compassion which impacts on thoughts and feelings and, in the safety of gentle practice, the client can begin to imbue the practice with kindness and observe the changes that this creates. Over time, this may well be introduced into daily life and impact on their relationship with themselves and others.

The more that mindfulness is practised, the greater the capacity to familiarise oneself with the internal experiences of the body, heart and mind. This then leads to a deeper, more compassionate awareness of the whole self.

The relationship between mindfulness and compassion

Repeatedly at conferences and so on, I hear from mindfulness teachers how self-compassion is inherent within mindfulness. I don't disagree with this, of course. From a non-secular perspective, this is certainly true. However, as more and more teachers and trainers are being taught to deliver secular mindfulness, the integrated quality of compassion has been lost, and the two separated out. Of course, the act of taking time to pay attention, to do a practice of any sort, is certainly, in itself, an act of self-compassion. It is also true to say that the more practice we do, the more we stimulate and develop the parts of the brain associated with self-compassion and compassion for others.

I do, however, think that, in a more secular context, teaching mindfulness alone can be dry and unfulfilling, rather like eating a rice cracker. I'm sure it is also a contributory factor to some of the backlash around mindfulness teaching of late, in that paying attention in the moment is of significant benefit but it does not necessarily give you the tools to take you forwards.

In the West, the recent trend has been to view mindfulness and compassion as separate entities, so this book sets out to explain the relationship between the two and restore balance in understanding and teaching, returning to a more wholesome and rounded appreciation of the power inherent within the relationship between mindfulness and compassion.

Mindful awareness is certainly the key to everything. Without this we have no way of knowing how to choose the best way to move forwards, to change and create new opportunities for ourselves. The relationship between mindfulness and compassion, therefore, is that mindfulness helps us to develop awareness, enabling us to tune in to whatever is arising for us in the present moment; and then, by bringing an attitude of compassion, wise action can begin, leading to change.

The teacher is inviting the client to cut through the constant, mindless habits, which come about from living life on autopilot, simply by becoming aware. This, however, is just the tip of the iceberg. The client may then be invited to explore what is truly present, bringing attention to all aspects of their being, their thought patterns, emotional tone and physical sensations in the body. This can lead to a feeling of extreme vulnerability when one really sees oneself in the raw, turning towards all the experiences in the moment, including the difficult ones. This is often where mindfulness teachers stop and invite their clients to just "be" with these experiences, however painful. Without question there is merit in this, creating the conditions for open, radical acceptance, spaciousness and change. However, if we *only* have mindful awareness, it may well be that to shield ourselves from the pain of distressing circumstances we just put our defence layers back on and recreate a shell to retreat into. This response is both unhealthy and unhelpful.

The question, often subconsciously, arises: "What can I do with what I am experiencing?" Mindfulness is clearly not the full answer to this question; compassion is. Compassion creates an environment for calming the nervous system through self-soothing, repeating self-comforting phrases such as "It's not your fault", and giving oneself the tools to choose to move forwards in a new, less harsh and less combative way.

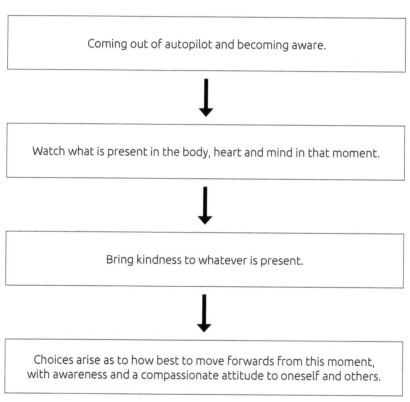

Figure 1.1 *The relationship between mindfulness and compassion.*

Compassion can help to change the relationship with who we are, what we do and what we feel, and to think about ourselves, other people, our situation and the stories that we have created about ourselves and our lives before now and into the future.

Feeling vulnerable can help to support us in developing new pathways and new ways of living our lives, by seeing things in perspective, creating changes and letting go of the things that don't support us. In this way we can build new experiences and create more opportunities and new relationships with things and people that enable us to feel fulfilled. When we try out these new ways of being and these new ways of seeing, the feeling can be quite excruciating – we can really squirm and it can feel so alien – but that's where mindfulness comes in again. Being aware of those sensations, sitting with those sensations and going deeper into those sensations creates more resources to investigate this more self-compassionate approach to life.

By peeling back the layers more and more, one can begin to experience the more subtle and nuanced thinking and feeling patterns that are no longer supportive. One can experiment with what it's like to be kind and even kinder, and notice how that feels. One then becomes more aware of the rewards and benefits that help to support growth and develop transformation to a new place of being, with softness and kindness at every step promoting equanimity and ease.

Anchoring inquiry

When teaching a practice, the teacher sets the intention to facilitate the client in paying attention with different attitudes: namely compassion, non-judgement, non-striving and curiosity.

Intentions and motivations

Sometimes it can feel as if inquiry is arbitrary and that the teacher is simply asking a question and waiting to see what feedback they get. However, the teacher is not trying to find out *why* something happened, as perhaps would be the case in other interventions; instead they're asking open-ended questions to explore *what* happened.

Knowing and then setting the intention or motivation for guiding a practice will help with this exploration or unfolding of experiences during inquiry, asking questions related to the practice intentions.

Each practice may have a slightly different intention: for example, the intention to place attention on different parts of the body in stillness, such as the body scan; and then again in movement, as in a mindful movement practice; and then observing the different experiences between the two practices, even though the object of attention, the body, is the same.

When a teacher holds intentionality in mind, the inquiry process can pivot around these intentions so that there is some focus. Specific questions relating to these intentions and the effect of the attitude within the practice on the ability to remain aligned with the intention may support a deepening of the client's understanding during inquiry.

1.
The teacher sets the intention/motivation for teaching a particular practice, either for themselves or explaining the intention to clients, if appropriate.

2.
The teacher guides the practice, dropping in small pearls of language relating to those intentions/motivations throughout.

3.
The teacher structures some of the inquiry questions around these intentions/motivations.

Figure 1.2 Inquiry sequence.

Imagine, for example, that the teacher has just started to see a client who suffers with anxiety as a result of feeling that they're always moving from one thing to another. Teaching a short practice focusing on the breath may well be a good place to start. The teacher may therefore guide the client through the practice as follows:

1.
Teacher setting intention with the client to be present in this moment:
"What is sometimes helpful with mindfulness is that it
gives us the opportunity to drop into the present moment,
giving space to simply 'be' in the busyness of the day."

2.
Teacher guiding practice:
"As we sit here in this moment, rest your attention on the
sensations of the body breathing, being aware in this moment
of how it feels as the breath comes in and out of the body."

3.
Teacher leading inquiry:
"By bringing your attention to the sensations of the breath,
were you able to sense into the experience in the moment?"
"What was it like for you to pay attention to the
breath as it came in and out of the body?"

Figure 1.3 Inquiry on a short practice.

Core features

These intentions are often synonymous with the core features of mindfulness, and by maintaining an awareness of these features, a familiar anchor from which to conduct the whole process of inquiry is formulated.

A client's specific presenting problem does not have a correlated specific practice; so, for example, if a client is suffering with anxiety, there is no specific practice to help alleviate this anxiety. However, becoming familiar with the rationale for teaching specific practices can assist in relating inquiry to the core features pertinent to that specific practice.

The core features can be viewed as golden threads that run throughout inquiry, starting with the building of understanding of what mindfulness is in a simple, accessible way. These threads then run through each session, each time widening, deepening and expanding, making them more relevant as learning through experiences, dialogue and practical applications leads to them becoming more embedded over time.

Reconnecting with the child within

With the recent upsurge of interest in mindfulness, some people think it has only been around for a decade or so and view the teaching of new skills as a laborious process of putting effort into learning. It's true that it can sometimes feel like this at the outset, but it soon starts to feel as if there's a sense of reconnection with the innate sense of self and being true to inherent core values and beliefs.

In fact, the vast majority of us were born with the ability to be mindful. One only needs to think back to childhood and the pleasure gained from playing and being creative, and the instant joy at seeing or experiencing something fully in the moment. This is what we are reconnecting with, although many people feel this capacity is beyond their grasp as they're caught up with ruminating about past experiences, worrying about what tomorrow may bring, thinking about the same things over and over, revisiting conversations, replaying events and wishing things could be different.

A teacher's role is to support others in revitalising these innate skills, allowing them to resurface by teaching the core features of training attention and awareness, taking the client out of autopilot and, through the creation of space, enabling perspective to be regained. It is through the person's ability to become aware of the relationship between their thoughts, emotions and physical sensations, that they can see their habitual tendencies (usually developed in childhood in response to parenting and conditioning). This then gives them the freedom to choose to do things differently from now on, resulting in a sense of empowerment, resilience and resourcefulness.

Creating a safe space for exploration

During a Process of Inquiry workshop in 2018 I taught a compassionate mindful practice. After a comment from a participant in which she explained how the practice had helped, I reflected back to her:

> It sounds like the practice helped you to feel more safe, secure and OK with whatever was arising for you within every moment. Is this something that feels very familiar to you: that relationship between the changing sensations that you experienced in the practice and how you're able to be in your life?

When she had confirmed this was most definitely her experience, I went on to explain:

> If we learn, during the safety of practice, that things are constantly changing and we become accustomed to this, then we know too that when facing problems in life, in a few moments, hours, days or months this will be very different and this can be an anchoring and grounding experience. We don't get caught up in aversion and resistance, which adds to our suffering, but allow the space and time for the events to unfold in their own way.

My comments had the effect of contextualising and validating the experiences she had already felt but not verbalised, giving the concept more clarity and instilling the benefits of practice more fully. She now knew that she could identify patterns in the safety of practice, which could lead to a rounder appreciation of how this enhances every-day life.

When I am assessing students who are training to become teachers, at the end of the practice I often hear them saying, "Now come back into the room from wherever you were." I explain that teachers should be encouraging clients to stay very firmly in the room, anchored with their bodily sensations to the present-moment experiences. If this is difficult – it can be overwhelming when emotions become activated – I suggest advising the clients to use their sensory perception through sight, smell, taste or hearing, thereby externalising the sensations, This has the effect of calming the nervous system and regaining equilibrium.

During inquiry a client may explain that they lost concentration as they became emotional. The teacher can ask questions such as: "What did you do when you started to feel overwhelmed with your emotions?" This helps to build resources to enable the client to feel more anchored in subsequent practices.

Myth-busting

A teacher needs to clarify that it's not always appropriate to be mindful. Teaching discernment as to when and to what extent it's helpful to be mindful is part of any training. It's a choice to make in any moment, which has the effect of being liberating. The majority of clients who attend mindfulness sessions bring with them learning from the past, as well as plans for the future. If a teacher is not explicit, some clients believe that the intention is to be mindful all of the time, which is extremely challenging.

My father has Alzheimer's disease and I know first-hand how catastrophic it is to only live in the moment, not remembering or being able to bring learning from his past into the present and having no concept of what his future may hold. It makes everyday tasks that should be simple, complex, as he has to relearn everything in every moment. However, I also observe how happy he is, having had to relinquish all memories of what his life was like before and having no capacity to make plans or decisions about the future. I know this isn't the experience of all those suffering with a form of dementia and that this too is a state of impermanence. I can, therefore, only speak from personal experience when I say that he is a more mellow, accepting and loving human being than he was when he had all his faculties.

Practice

As we have already explored, the inquiry process gives us the opportunity to enter into a dialogue about the experiences that arose during and in response to practice, but what does "practice" actually mean?

When I use the term "practice", I think of a setting of intention to create a space, allowing the movement and acknowledgement of thoughts, feelings and sensations to arise. It's rather like a vast ocean where experiences rise to the surface, often unbidden, precipitating a ripple on the surface of the ocean. These experiences are then enfolded back into the expanse of water, allowing others to arise into the sunlight. Throughout, we can hold an awareness of this process with a kindly attitude, trusting the process and observing the experiences with a sense of curiosity. Mindfulness practice is supported by a state of alertness and clarity of mind, enabling the meditator to be more sharply attentive to the object.

One of my teachers, Andy Wistreich,[4] explained to me that, during practice, which can be likened to a still pond, a little fish of awareness comes in to see what's happening within the practice, gently investigating into the small crevices, without disturbing the practice itself. I find this analogy quite helpful as sometimes I have noticed that awareness can precipitate thinking, which inevitably alters my experiences of practice. The fish of awareness is so small that it doesn't disturb "the water" of the practice in any way.

Shorter practices

A teacher will often introduce clients to mindfulness by teaching them shorter practices. It is such a good place to start, akin to training muscles in a gym, where starting with shorter practices and smaller weights helps to build stamina slowly over time. These mindfulness practices include those that support coming into the present moment. This could be through an awareness of the body, such as feeling into the sensations of the feet on the floor and giving the weight of the body up to gravity, or perhaps an abdominal breathing practice, or a breathing space or awareness of sounds practice. All of these are helpful in teaching us that we have a choice about how, when and where to place our attention in any given moment. This helps to build an appreciation that, through choice, we can decide whether to be mindful, anchored in the here and now, rather than constantly buffeted around by events and other people; it creates an oasis of calm and a chance to recalibrate and be restful, even if only for a few moments. A sense of stability, equanimity and ease can start to be developed in response to these shorter practices.

Longer practices

I always think of longer practices as being 20 minutes or more in duration, supporting the neurological changes that will be explored in Chapter 3. This can be a formal or longer meditation practice such

---

4   Personal communication (2019) with Andy Wistreich (Buddhist teacher).

as a body scan, mindful movement or mindful breathing practice. The client is invited to rest their attention on a specific object, noticing their mind wandering over and over again, and bringing it back as many times as it wanders. This is real brain training and is something to build over time: the building of the mental muscle. This leads to a host of benefits, including better clarity, concentration and an ability to keep perspective. A colleague, Angie Ward,[5] was telling me recently how mindfulness training has helped her enormously in choosing to "switch off" when she's at home, that is, not thinking about work or what she's got to do when she returns. She explained how, on reflection, since learning mindfulness, her sleep is substantially better and her capacity to be present, wherever she is, has enhanced her life no end. When she's at work, she doesn't think about home, and vice versa.

Coping strategies

When a client becomes more aware of feelings of stress and anxiety, specific practices or techniques can be taught to cut through the automatic fight and flight responses, to bring about a greater sense of calm and ease and regain a feeling of control.

A simple but very effective coping strategy is the STOP technique.

S stands for stop whatever you are doing, as long as it is safe to do so.
T relates to taking attention to the body breathing, in particular abdominal breathing.
O is the really mindful part of the practice, observing the thoughts, feelings and sensations arising in that moment.
P is where you return/proceed to doing what you were doing, but with a mindful awareness.

Figure 1.4 STOP coping strategy.

Mindfulness contributes profoundly to the capacity to self-regulate and promote self-care, thereby creating an environment which supports a sense of being able to cope more readily.

---

5   Personal communication (2019) with Angie Ward (mindfulness and compassion teacher and trainer).

Daily activities

For me a significant part of what mindfulness meditation can do is the ability to bring a meditative approach to life's experiences in any moment one chooses. This is directly developed in response to the brain-training skill derived from practice, folding the practice into life. As with practice, I encourage clients to start with smaller, less demanding, shorter tasks and then increase them as their confidence and capacity grow.

Whilst doing a mundane task, the mind has a propensity to make up stories and imaginings or go into planning mode, thinking about all the jobs that still need to be done. In actual fact, these familiar activities (for example, doing the washing up, having a shower, brushing one's teeth, drinking a cup of tea, eating dinner, digging the garden) require little thought. By dropping into the present moment, it is possible to derive more pleasure from an experience (for example, feeling the warm water when showering, smelling the scent of the soap and hearing the water flowing from the shower head to the body and down the plug). It creates space and attention to the finer details, as does practice. The more this skill is developed, the greater the capacity to widen it out into more complex tasks such as during a conversation, driving, studying a document or writing a book!

By being able to live each moment, rather than ruminating about the past or pre-living the future before it's even arrived, which can lead to a sense of feeling overloaded and overwhelmed, the joy and richness of experiences in the here and now contribute profoundly to the experience of increased happiness.

A teacher has a role here in supporting the client to appreciate the relationship between practice and bringing an enhanced awareness to their daily life. This is achieved through inquiry. Exploring what happens in the client's mind and how it feels in the body and emotionally when being present during daily activities, and encouraging them to journal these experiences and to reflect on them later in the day or week, can bring about significant change and enhance their life boundlessly.

Why practice?

Whilst anchoring the inquiry in the core features of mindfulness through the combined approach of embodiment and verbalisation of the practice, one can start to become familiar with how the mind works by shining a light on the tendencies of the mind, which are often not in one's conscious awareness but inform everything on a subconscious level. Through the act of identifying the experience and naming the thoughts, emotions and physical sensations, one starts to bring these experiences to the conscious mind. This begins the process of seeing habitual patterns, through paying attention, and is usually reflected in the interactions in life and relationships. For example, one may become impatient with the practice, be anxious about whether it's being done right, or be annoyed with oneself or the teacher. Perhaps there's a tendency in life to be quite reactive, only to regret the subsequent actions when one has cooled down.

By exploring these common patterns, one can get to know oneself more intimately. This creates the platform for either acknowledging the helpful patterns or changing them, leading to a greater sense of control and empowerment.

Chapter 2

THE ICEBERG MODEL OF COMPASSIONATE MINDFUL INQUIRY

The benefits of a framework

After taking part in the Process of Inquiry workshop with me, one of my students, Gill,[1] commented that she now feels that she knows this territory as a result of exploring the model and appreciates that once she has familiarised herself with this process over time when teaching, she'll be able to let go of consciously following the model. Gill, a social worker, explains that having a sequence of questions to ask at each stage will augment her natural curiosity about what people are thinking and feeling and it will enhance her work, which necessitates developing a deeper understanding of the service user's emotional, physical and psychological status, right now.

The framework, therefore, has a role in helping a teacher to see the bigger picture and in developing their knowledge around the general direction to take from the outset. It includes some specific reference points and suggestions about how to get started and the best ways to proceed. It gives the whole process perspective, enabling more clarity around what the teacher is setting out to facilitate, giving the opportunity to plan, prioritise and pace teaching and learning.

Being a teacher of these practices is unlike most other teaching roles, where there is often some predictability, a right and a wrong answer and a general appreciation of what people will experience

---

1   Personal communication (2018) with Gill (social worker and mindfulness teacher).

when being taught a skill. Teaching mindfulness and compassion really isn't anything like this. Certainly, there are some general themes, feedback responses that occur quite frequently, and similarities as a result of certain practices. But this is very often not the case. I've been teaching these skills for 20 years and the reason I love it so much is that hearing about other people's experiences keeps it fresh and fascinating. I genuinely don't know what someone is going to say about their experience at any given moment. That is why it is so important that the teacher is anchored and centred when asking questions around experiences during practice. They need to have the confidence to "hold" whatever arises and know what to do and say in unpredictable circumstances.

Becoming familiar with a framework provides a safe haven, a comfort zone to revert to, so that the teacher can re-orientate inquiry with their client if things get a little uneasy and uncertain. Winging it and blindly continuing without a framework can not only result in teachers getting into difficulties and losing their way but, more importantly by far, the client may become uneasy or confused and, in the worst case scenario, more problems can result.

Learning inquiry is hard – there's no question about it. Although some teachers have a natural affinity for it and a natural curiosity and are good listeners, there's more to it than this and it is certainly a steep learning curve. There is no substitute for practising guiding inquiry and developing skills through experience. However, becoming familiarised with a framework can help to get the process started. I always tell my students to "teach what you know" and this knowing has to be, to some extent, from their own experience of practice and self-inquiry, particularly at the beginning. However, this experiential learning can also be profoundly enhanced with cognitive learning, which helps a teacher to grow the edges of their comfort zone and become more spontaneous and flexible within the wider context of the framework.

During a recent supervision session, a student sheepishly asked me if it was OK to enjoy the process of inquiry. She explained what a mutually rewarding experience it had seemed to be and found it deeply moving and energising. Her timid question made me laugh. This is the joyous side of this work: supporting others and resonating with them so that everyone benefits!

The core stages

Here, the core stages look like individual components and will be discussed as such, taking a look at one at a time. Consideration is given to their relevance in relation to both mindfulness and compassion.

The full model then sets out to explore more comprehensively how these core stages relate and inter-relate with one another, being at the centre of guiding practices and inquiry throughout.

Arising from these three core stages are the corresponding and sequential processes that are experienced in response to practice. Once these processes are better understood, they provide a framework for inquiry, enabling the teacher to appreciate how a client's understanding and experiences develop over time. Each process correlates to the neurological changes that occur, and they are fully explained, one at a time, in Chapter 3.

Figure 2.1 The core stages.

Paying attention
Mindfulness

As we have already investigated, the first core stage to the inquiry process consists of the development of awareness through paying attention. There's a paradox here in that we know that mindfulness practice develops self-awareness but we also know that a person has to be self-aware to know that they need mindfulness. By becoming aware of the effects of mindfulness and what happens when this is imbued with compassion, a deeper appreciation of how to approach life's challenges and initiate change is learnt and experienced. Practising mindfulness and noticing what is happening in the here and now (*direct* noticing) is just the start. Go deeper.

Compassion

By paying attention to the effects of mindfulness and what happens when this is imbued with compassion, a deeper appreciation of how to approach life's challenges and initiate change is learnt and experienced.

Reflective dialogue
Mindfulness

In the second core stage, reflective dialogue investigates noticing what happens when we pay attention to experiences. This is essential in developing more resources and understanding.

Compassion

This stage also reflects on what happens when we bring compassion to these experiences, creating some stability and kindness, as questions arise.

Linking
Mindfulness

The third core stage, linking the observations of the effects of awareness and what happens when the client notices these effects, enables the client to integrate their newfound knowledge and experience of the power of mindfulness and compassion to all aspects of their life.

Compassion

This core stage also links mindfulness and compassion, allowing scope for change, with kindness. *Now let's explore the inter-relationship of these core stages, and the processes arising from them, in more detail.*

The six processes of the Iceberg Model

For many years I have been working with the core stages, as set out above, but felt that a model that clarified the explicit and sequential relationship between mindfulness and compassion, in conjunction with these core stages and the processes arising from these stages, would be most helpful for the students and teachers of mindfulness. I wanted to devise a model that reflected my own personal experience of mindfulness and compassion and resonated with my professional experiences with clients. As often happens in life, having put in hours and hours of thinking about it, and after innumerable sketches and failed attempts at creating something clear and succinct, the idea then came to me in a flash whilst I was sitting on a train looking out of the window at the passing Somerset countryside. On that very same day, my designer suggested that I change MindfulnessUK's branding image to resemble an iceberg! It was an extraordinary synchronicity and one not to be ignored.

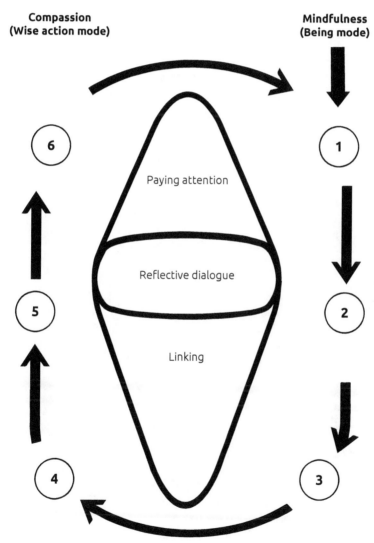

Figure 2.2 The Iceberg Model of Compassionate Mindful Inquiry (framework).

This is called the Iceberg Model, as developing awareness through paying attention is just the tip of the iceberg and there is so much more beneath the surface than meets the eye. The lower portion of the model is larger than the upper portion, depicting the vast amount of neurological and behavioural changes that manifest, in response to increased longevity, quantity and quality of practice, and the subsequent development of awareness, attention-training and emotional regulation that results.

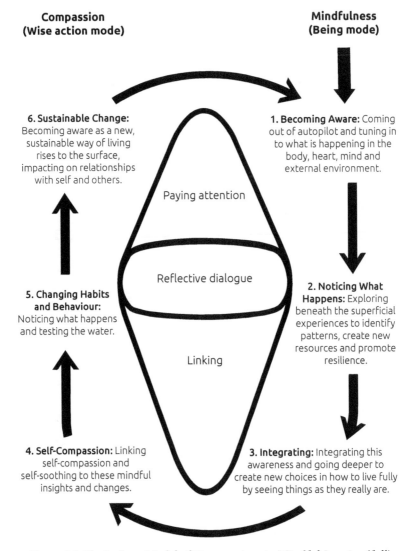

Figure 2.3 The Iceberg Model of Compassionate Mindful Inquiry (full)

Process 1: Becoming aware

The cycle begins in the top right when a teacher introduces mindfulness to their client. In essence, what the teacher is encouraging their client to pay attention to what arises when they stop, come out of autopilot and tune into their experiences in the present moment. This has to be the beginning: developing the skills to come out of doing mode, shift to being, and transfer their attention from their external experiences to their internal ones – their physical sensations, emotions and thoughts – whilst remaining open to everything within their whole field of awareness.

Training attention is where we start with all meditation practices. This ability to bring the mind back, over and over again, whilst anchoring the attention on an object (for example, the breath), has profound benefits. Developing this capacity to become attentive is imperative before proceeding more deeply with practice.

To be clear, it is not asking people to simply sit still and be quiet with an upright spine. Although this posture can certainly be beneficial, it is not actually that special – even animals have the capacity to do it (think of a bird or a monkey sitting on a tree branch). We humans, however, are unique in that our brains have developed the ability to pause and consciously choose what we pay attention to; and the more we exercise this mental muscle, the more profound the benefits are neurologically.

The first process also explores *direct* noticing about what happened during the practice in relation to physical sensations such as touch, breath, sounds, colours, textures, to the emotional experiences, as well as thoughts. The body is akin to a barometer, providing information as to how one is feeling in the moment, as it is the place where emotions and experiences of anxiety and tension are stored. The body processes information from the brain and emotions more slowly, so this is where clues as to how one is actually experiencing life reside.

Much of my clinical work has been in supporting people who have been abused or traumatised in some way. They often disconnect from their physical sensations as they feel overwhelmed by the information stored in their body. Sometimes, therefore, it is helpful to begin by paying attention to external experiences, such as the air touching the skin or sensations in the extremities (for example, the toes), or further away still (for example, distant sounds). As confidence and familiarity build, residual, stored experiences can be explored and the body can become a place of abiding safety and refuge.

This is the stage where awareness starts to build and attention is trained so that the client can start to become acquainted with the full nature of their experiences in any given moment.

It is important that the teacher retains an open mind, asking open questions to ensure there is no expectation or imputation from the teacher as to what "should" have been experienced. A few years ago I met a client, Helen, who experienced physical sensations as colours and smells, so I gave her the space to describe what she noticed in her own words, not interjecting or asking her to explain anything in more detail. She had a delightfully clear appreciation of her own experiences without me constraining them by asking her to explain them in another way in order for me to understand them better.

In addition to inquiring about physical sensations, the teacher also asks about emotions or feelings and any thoughts that might have arisen during the practice, often in relation to where these are experienced in the body. Questions around these experiences will help the client to become more aware of what happened, serving to step back from the immersion in experiences and witness them as an observer.

In this way too, the opportunity to switch on the parasympathetic nervous system arises: the rest and digest part of the nervous system, which, as will be explored in Chapter 3, stimulates the relaxation response. Of course, this is of profound benefit and is often the experience of those who prefer to do shorter practices, perhaps using apps and cherry-picking mindfulness tools as a way of coping with everyday stresses. Without doubt this can have significant benefits and contributes to a feeling of resilience and empowerment.

However, using these skills in isolation does not create fundamental and sustainable brain changes or a relational awareness of us as complex human beings, the benefits being quite superficial and short-lived in nature. If the extent of one's practice is coming into the present moment to elicit a sense of calm, it can act as something of a sticking plaster to feel better right now. I see it as a bit of a seesaw: the seat goes down when one feels bad, and the practice helps to balance things out again in that moment, short-term. However, the effect remains superficial and without substance, and the seat will drop down again soon enough if one returns to old habits in thoughts and behaviour. The seat can only remain balanced and in equilibrium in response to longer term practice.

There's potential for a discussion here around cause and effect. These practices are dealing with the effects of stresses that have been experienced but they do not address the cause. There is a sense, therefore, of a disconnect between the practices and life in that they're layered on top to help the person cope but the scope for building more robust foundations is not realised, thereby stabilising the seesaw's seats.

Therefore, it's an essential place to start, but there's so much further to go, deepening into the awareness that arises through practice to elicit fundamental changes that impact on the causes of stress.

Many years ago I taught the Mindfulness-Based Stress Reduction (MBSR) programme to a cohort that all worked together quite closely. I spent the majority of the course staying with this process, as the clients were so disassociated from their physical sensations – their experiences in the here and now – that it was helpful to take the time to centre them, to tune into this moment. If I had gone too swiftly towards the next processes, it would have been too cognitive, and they would not have reaped the benefits they did. By staying focused on their current experiences in their body, as a group they learnt a tremendous amount around the choices they made at work and how they were all constantly suffering high levels of exhaustion and burn-out by not attending to their own direct needs (for example, when they were thirsty, hungry, needed a break or would benefit from some support from their manager or colleagues). By learning to de-centre, step away from being immersed in their work and become more like witnesses to their experiences, they were able to make healthier, deeper choices, thereby enabling them to sustain their role to the benefit of themselves and those they were caring for in a more wholesome way.

I would always start guiding any practice by developing the client's capacity to become more aware, tuning into the feelings associated with the transition from our external world to our internal world and the busyness of getting there (for example, watching hesitation or resistance to change focus or the urges to speed up this process). Taking the time to go through the process can often facilitate a sense of "coming home to the body", back to the familiarity of now.

Teaching clients to become aware of the posture through specific teaching cues, the sensations of the ground beneath them, the movement of the body with the breath, and the experiences in the spine, shoulders, hands, neck, head and face, as well as the space without and within, creates a place of equanimity for whatever practice is to come. This development of a "holding" space is profoundly beneficial, allowing a sense of safety to be developed to permit deeper experiences to bubble up to the surface.

Inquiry also has the effect of enabling a client to learn and explore the language in relation to their experiences. For example, a client who is suffering with a painful knee might say after a practice, "My leg was painful because...", and then go into the story involving an incident, regrets, anger, catastrophising, or whatever. As the client builds awareness, becomes more attuned and begins to inter-relate experiences more proficiently, they may say, "I noticed my leg was painful and that makes me feel less confident about myself, which has the effect of stopping me saying yes to things as often as I'd like to."

I am often told by clients that their partner, relative or friend is really laid back, and the assumption is that they are therefore very mindful. People have the capacity to be really unperturbed by life's difficulties but this does not necessarily mean that they are aware. It may be that they take time out to "be in the moment" but actually they may be zoned out, disconnected or desensitised to the full range of experiences in that moment. This can certainly be very helpful at times, particularly if one has a history of trauma, but it is not necessarily a mindful state that they're in.

So, whilst it is imperative to develop awareness first as there's so much learning here, once a capacity to tune into present moment experiences has been learnt, clients are able to experience the subsequent processes, whilst still maintaining their ability to stay connected.

Being mindful can sometimes feel quite effortful and perturbing, creating a sense of wobbliness, so clients need support in continuing with this process. The teacher must guide them gently and with kindness as they continue to practice and their brain starts to change.

EXAMPLES OF QUESTIONS

Ask questions to help the client become more aware of their physical sensations, using their senses, including their mind, tuning into their direct experiences. The body provides an important source of information about whether the client is tense, stressed, lethargic, etc. However, for some people, the body can be quite elusive, experiencing little from the neck downwards, and clients can slip into a narrative or story about their experiences, so the teacher needs to guide questions accordingly.

What did you notice inside your body?

Be more specific: What were your physical sensations, including sounds, feelings, colours, textures, movement, smells and temperature?

Did you notice if you felt your emotions in your body? Please describe these if you can.

What emotions did you feel in your body and did these sensations change?

Were you aware of what was happening with your thoughts?

Were there any sensations associated with your thoughts: worry, tension, wanting to move on, butterflies?

What was it like to come out of autopilot and drop into the present moment?

What are you experiencing right now as a result of describing those experiences?

What were those experiences like for you, if you don't mind me asking?

Process 2: Noticing what happens

When we notice what happens when we pay attention, we are exploring beneath the superficial experiences to identify patterns, create new resources and promote resilience. By then proceeding to the second core stage of reflective dialogue, the process arising can precipitate the client can start to investigate thoughts, actions, emotional patterns, urges, resistance and reactivity at a deeper level, creating an environment for learning and change.

This dialogue around the experiences helps the client to place the direct noticing into a personal context by exploring how it felt, what they did, and their reactions to their mind wandering, for example. By developing this skill, the client can begin to recognise patterns and responses to their experiences. It is valuable to recognise patterns and explore whether the act of bringing awareness to them actually has an impact, potentially creating change.

Dialogue also provides an opportunity and safe environment in which to begin to turn towards or lean into difficulties and suffering. By exploring what happens, a client can begin to see maladaptive behaviours and coping responses and start to appreciate that maybe these are no longer as supportive as they used to be, perhaps having been developed during childhood or in previous relationships.

Unlike therapeutic interventions that give instructions for changes to be made (for example, saying a positive affirmation or asking someone to relax), here a client can appreciate that the act of paying attention elicits change without them having tried to make it happen. This is exciting because all one needs to do is hold present-moment experiences with attention, accepting things as they really are, and something almost magical happens: change happens on its own. For example, feelings of discomfort ebb and flow, and pain can dissipate, or at least change in nature and severity.

One doesn't have to go too deeply into quantum physics to learn about the "observer effect". Lynne McTaggart (2003) discusses how this term means that the act of observing will influence the phenomenon being observed.

I often think that this is what is happening here during this process: bringing to conscious awareness what actually happens during the first stage of observation and noting how this precipitates change, unbidden.

The client needs to have been made to feel safe initially for this more subtle appreciation of the impermanent nature of experiences to be noticed, felt and observed to the full. A teacher can use analogies here to give the client opportunities to appreciate these changing sensations (for example, inviting them to see thoughts passing by like clouds in the sky, a leaf on a stream or whether to get off the train at the station).

Teachers can suggest that there's comfort to be derived from paying attention to areas of discomfort and pain with a sense of curiosity, then sensing into these changing sensations and intensities to observe and take on board more fully that nothing is static.

As humans we often try very hard to keep things as they are. However, when we become more accustomed to the small changes in our experiences, we are not so dislodged by the more significant changes in our lives and are able to keep more of a sense of equilibrium and equanimity.

In essence, the client is encouraged to reflect on their experiences in relation to what they have noticed. It is here that the teacher can encourage exploration, expansion and validation by inviting them to be more descriptive of their experiences, clarifying what happened, what it felt like and inquiring more deeply with an authentic curiosity.

When the client begins to be able to identify direct experiences and these start to become familiar, there is an opportunity then to explore the relationship between these experiences and the effect they're having. Awareness of the experiences of the body has the response of promoting connectivity and can be considered as a window to the mind by developing an understanding of the relationship between the body, emotions and mind.

Identifying and describing thoughts builds awareness of the difference between the doing and being modes of the mind so that the client can inquire into the nature of their patterns. It opens them up to the possibility of using the practice as a first step for coping with difficult thoughts. More appreciation of tendencies to dwell in the past or anticipate the future arises here. Learning that by choosing to observe thoughts one has the capacity to control them is insightful. It contributes to the loosening of attachment by stepping back from the entanglement of thoughts, physical feelings and emotions to create space and develop a sense of control and greater perspective.

It can also narrow the angle of attention. By focusing, for example, on the tangible experience of the breath (perhaps with the question "What happened to your thoughts as you focused on your breath?"), one can appreciate how to interrupt and disengage from mental activity.

By bringing attention to the emotional tone, a teacher can encourage a tuning in to what is, and then a realisation that one has a choice to not become too attached to the emotional experience.

Staying attuned to a client's body language is crucial. If they are closed and protective, the teacher must discern whether to let them be and not expose their vulnerabilities, or to support them through soft, gentle inquiry questions to create a sense of opening up to their experiences.

EXAMPLES OF QUESTIONS

What would it be like for you to describe what you noticed during the practice?

How did you feel when your mind wandered?

What did you do with your wandering mind and how did that feel emotionally?

Did bringing awareness to your thoughts change your experience?

Is there a specific phrase within the practice that touched you?

What happened to these experiences through paying attention? Did they change or not?

Is there a familiar pattern emerging here?

Can you say how that experience unfolded?

Were you able to notice how that felt in your body and did this change during the practice?

How did it feel to notice the fluctuating and changing sensations, the impermanent nature of your experiences?

Were you aware of a relationship between your thoughts, emotions and body?

Do you feel differently now at the end of the practice compared with how you did at the beginning? Can you say a little more about how that is for you right now?

Process 3: Integrating

As the client deepens their awareness of their experiences, they are able to link the experiences, link the processes thus far and integrate this learning directly into their lives. Sometimes this can elicit a real "light bulb" moment in which this unveiling of understanding can lead to a broader sense of perspective and appreciation of their true reality.

Once the client has started to become more familiar with their habitual tendencies, they can begin to deepen their mindful awareness still further, investigating how their changing understanding of themselves and how they relate to others can be linked to the core features of mindfulness and how these can support life outside meditation. I often think of meditation as being a place where every aspect of an experience is magnified and thus it gives a comfortable and safe space to take a look at what's going on with truthfulness and honesty. When this becomes familiar and feels authentic, one can then start to integrate what has been learnt into the choices made about how to live, starting small and being kind around the changes that have been chosen.

This also precipitates a capacity to link the present with the past and future, obviating the need for analysis. For example, noticing that there's a sense of anxiety in the present through an awareness of irritation in the body; then, rather than getting caught up in a cyclical anxiety vortex, whereby one becomes anxious that one will be anxious, observing that the anxiety is arising because of a background worry about the exam tomorrow; then, a choice is presented, such as study further, have a rest, exercise or practice.

Sensing into the capacity to open up to choices, where perhaps there was a perception that no choices were available, will help the client to link back into their practice too. The teacher helps the client to see that the value of practice far exceeds sitting quietly watching the breath.

Society presents us with so many challenges that sometimes we can get drawn towards these external demands of our time and energy, the external pleasures and attachment to satisfaction. This can happen for so long and to such an extent that we can end up living our lives far removed from the things that create inner peace and harmony. Through this process it is possible to begin to help clients to reconnect with their core beliefs and inner values, as the onion layers of distraction and defence are peeled away to reveal what is truly there, what really matters. Living life congruently and authentically in this way leads to more of a sense of ease through non-striving and a feeling of connectivity with others on a fundamental level.

Therefore, as awareness and understanding build, the skilled teacher can start to link the client's learning from the practice to a wider context, exploring how mindfulness can help to cut through cyclical patterns, enhance daily life and deepen understanding about the self and relationships with others.

During this process, the teacher can link much of what a client has experienced through practice and inquiry to their everyday life, in a practical way. This may include an exploration of how to link the core features, the attitudes and/or benefits of mindfulness to the choices they make – for example, their behaviour and relationships.

An understanding can now be developed in relation to the interconnected nature of experiences within themselves and their interpersonal relationships. There is often a shift here, moving from focusing on the self to seeing that we all share vulnerabilities, suffering, problems and difficulties in our lives – that sense of common humanity.

There is more of an opportunity to talk about how we can play with the edge of our comfort/discomfort and how this can be translated into our daily life. This leads to a greater sense of resilience and resourcefulness, knowing when it is appropriate to stay in the comfort zone and, at other times pushing the boundaries, knowing that the supportive foundations have been laid to underpin this place of unease and to choose to return to a place of safety when required.

I might introduce this concept through mindful movement. For example, asking the client to extend their leg, bringing the toes towards them and experiencing the stretch in the back of the leg. Clients will automatically stop this stretch as they get to the edge of their comfort zone. I may then invite them to open into the back of their knee further, just beyond the natural stretch, and notice what it feels like to open up to a restriction. During inquiry I might then ask what it was like to create space in a place of restriction or to explore what happened as this position was held. The stretch reflex usually softens the stretch after 20 seconds or so and this is a good analogy for what happens in other areas of a client's experience: staying with an uncomfortable experience can result in softening and accepting it rather than pushing against it.

Thus, the clients learn how to embed mindfulness into life's experiences, facilitating an integration of the attitudes learnt into daily life so that it becomes routine. For some, the transition from meditation to daily life evolves naturally, whilst for others a teacher may need to hold the space for clients to find their own connections. It is often tempting to teach the point, but the client must experience it for themselves in order to gain insight and transformation.

EXAMPLES OF QUESTIONS

What does it feel like for you to notice what happens when you pay attention?

Can you identify your experience with other areas of your life – your relationships, for example?

By linking your direct experiences and having developed an understanding of how that relates to your thoughts, feelings and sensations, do you have a sense that you could do things differently in the future?

Now that you have identified some of your patterns, do you feel more able to make different choices as a result?

How could you transfer what you have learnt through this practice to benefit your life?

Does your experience resonate with your core beliefs? Can you see how you can connect with these more readily moving forwards?

How does bringing in one of the attitudes affect your experiences?

That sounds like a real shift for you. Is there anything else you'd like to explore in relation to what you've just noticed?

How does it feel right now to describe what you have discovered about yourself?

Process 4: Self-compassion

This is where one truly shifts into the need for self-compassion, moving from training the attention, seeing things as they really are, to the next phase of construction and wise action. Mindfulness helps one to gain clarity, but what does one do with that newfound knowledge, a state that can sometimes feel raw and be a place of vulnerability?

By bringing kindness to experiences, such as the breath, the sense of separation is reduced as clients move away from pure observation to a "felt sense". A question such as "What did you notice when you shifted from observation to feeling?" brings about that sense of connectivity between all aspects of the self, as well as resonating with the experiences of others.

Change is scary – believe me, I know. As humans, we like our routine, and like to know where we are and feel safe, but this often comes from a place of delusion, including patterns from the past that are now no longer relevant and stories we tell ourselves to perpetuate the delusion and keep up appearances. So, when we try out something new it can trigger anxiety, anger, frustration and other strong feelings of unease. This is where we need to shift, to be more compassionate to ourselves, to be more self-soothing and self-nurturing, to ensure that we don't simply revert to our comfortable, potentially damaging default position. Compassion builds the capacity, resources and resilience that enable us to move forwards in a new way now that we can see more clearly what's really going on.

In Chapter 1 I mentioned how building mental muscle through meditation practice is akin to building physical muscle in a gym. This analogy also applies to developing the muscle of kindness. One has to start off slowly, which can be a somewhat painful process, mainly because we're not used to the emotional sensations that can arise from this form of exercise. Just like going to the gym, the more we do it, the bigger and stronger this muscle gets until it becomes our new norm.

Although compassion has already started to develop, perhaps in an implicit way, through the act of practising mindfulness meditation, it is during this process that mindfulness and compassion are explicitly linked and integrated to begin to effect change internally through building new skills and techniques such as self-soothing.

Introducing self-compassion in this overt way can certainly feel very alien and make one squirm with awkwardness, but it's the beginning of a new way of relating to the self. For example, if a client says they are very self-critical, mindfulness helps them to identify this habit and to notice, when it arises, how it feels in the body and emotions as well as the resulting behaviour. But this is only part of the picture. By bringing in some self-soothing, the teacher gives the client something to "do" with these critical voices; for example, encouraging them to say something like, "It's OK to be thinking these things, sweetheart, but I now have resources, which means these thoughts no longer affect me as they used to. I realise that thoughts are not facts."

Asking clients what it would be like to treat themselves as they would their best friend if they were suffering in some way is often quite illuminating. Here the teacher is starting to introduce this as a concept, a way of changing the client's relationship with themselves from one of judgement and striving, to comfort and care. Sometimes the introduction of physical touch, such as inviting clients to place a hand on the heart, can help them engage with this approach more readily.

At the end of a mindful self-compassion retreat, participant Ali Pember[2] commented, quite emotionally:

> Although I know about the importance of caring for myself, it was wonderful to be reminded of the physical gesture of placing my hand on my heart – it was very soothing and allowed me to embody self-compassion in a way that conceptual thought could simply not achieve.

By beginning to develop the resources of self-compassion, one can feel more empowered to open up to the emotional climate within and know that if things become a little intense or overwhelming, one can always use mindfulness to come back to. Deciding to mindfully drink a cup of tea or take the attention away from the body can help to dampen feelings of emotional activation. In this way mindfulness supports emotional regulation and allows emotions to be explored from a position of mindful safety.

In this fourth process it becomes very clear that the teacher is helping the client to move from the art of just being (mindfulness), to doing something to support the integration of new skills through the development of a more compassionate attitude as a way of initiating change.

Lyubomirsky (2010) explains that three factors have the greatest influence on increasing our happiness. Firstly, there is the capacity to reframe the situation more positively. This is only possible, I believe, once a full appreciation of the true situation has been determined. Secondly, the ability to experience gratitude is profoundly important. When one has removed the veils of defences and started to reconnect with core beliefs, inner values and humanity, then one can experience

---

2   Personal communication (2019) with Ali Pember (mindfulness teacher).

gratitude in its purest form. Lastly, levels of happiness are based on the choices made to be kind and generous to both the self and others.

When leading inquiry with a client, the teacher can facilitate enhancement of their experiences in all three areas by supporting their capacity to investigate them from a different perspective, such as in the exercises around recording pleasant events and exploring what sustains and drains them, so they can make healthier choices. Helping them to investigate ways of being kinder through their practice and the impact this can have on how they communicate, behave and interact with themselves and others creates choices around opportunities to be more kind and generous.

Bethany, a client who suffered with excruciating chronic pain as a result of a freak accident caused by her colleague at work in which she lost her hand, started to feel better able to manage her condition as she saw me weekly one-to-one to learn mindfulness and compassion. After about four sessions she was practising mindfulness daily and, surprisingly to her, the pain resulting from neuroma around the site of trauma, her stump, started to subside. Although this is not always the case by any means, mindfulness can help a client to feel more in control in a gentler, less critical way, and pain can be ameliorated.

Bethany had suffered with pain for over ten years and began to recognise that she was somewhat habituated to this and the debilitating effect it had on her life physically, mentally and emotionally. She was beginning to bring kindness to herself and was noticing and then softening around the anger towards her ex-colleague that she had been holding on to for all this time. The overall effect of this change in attitude and being taught practices and coping strategies to utilise for her own benefit whenever she needed to was a change in physical sensations, creating more ease in her body.

This is such a good example of the inter-relationship between the body, thoughts and emotions; if a client is able to bring awareness and self-compassion to one aspect, there's potential for a healthy ripple effect to the rest of their experiences.

The fidelity of the core features and the attitudes of mindfulness can now be explored with understanding and kindness, giving rise to a deeper level of acceptance. This understanding of the value of accepting what is, and not trying to change or fix difficulties, contributes to the development of confidence, courage-building and resilience.

Having clear discussions regarding the role and value of compassion, teaching specific self-compassion practices and inquiring into the effects of these on the body, heart and mind can be powerful and transformative. It's important to help the client explore fully what it feels like to bring kindness and care to what they've observed about themselves throughout this process.

EXAMPLES OF QUESTIONS

How do you think it would feel to bring compassion in here?

If you did bring in self-compassion, did that change your experience within the practice?

Can you describe what it felt like to be compassionate to yourself when you noticed that?

What would it feel like to care for yourself as if you were a small child or your best friend?

Are there other opportunities in your life to bring in more kindness and, if so, how do you think that might change things for you?

What I (the teacher) have a sense of is that you were compassionate to yourself when you noticed that. Would you like to say a little bit about this?

Are you able to describe how you may be able to work with this going forwards?

What happens to your aversion, your resistance, when you bring in a little bit of kindness?

The teacher can recap the client's phrases to demonstrate how they were able to take care of themselves and validate their resourcefulness.

Process 5: Changing habits and behaviour

What happens here is that when change is experienced, however beneficial it might be, the client often simply doesn't like it – it's unfamiliar and harder work. Therefore, they may sabotage any progress by reverting to what they know, however damaging and life-limiting this may be. Often at this point it is helpful to take the intervention at a slower pace and introduce the concept and practices of self-compassion, mindfully identifying reactive and maladaptive behaviours.

The teacher is encouraging a client to test the water, try something new and different and then apply the second core stage (reflective dialogue) when habits are challenged and changed.

Through inquiry we can help clients to facilitate their understanding of the distinction between their primary feelings of pain, be they physical, psychological or emotional, and the secondary suffering that is evoked as a result of their response to their pain. Mindfulness has helped to create more of a place of stability and resourcefulness from which to investigate these distinctions and, as a client starts to make changes based on this new understanding, the teacher can enhance this progression through inquiring into how they can bring more kindness to these choices. In this way, clients are able to "turn into the skid" more readily. This is a great analogy for what the stage engenders – rather like a car that hits a patch of ice, counter-intuitively the driver is taught to turn into the spin and the car will stop. As difficulties arise, clients are taught to turn towards them, counter-intuitively, bringing kindness to this process.

The teacher's role is to promote dialogue around what happens when self-kindness and care are introduced, asking questions relating to what the client noticed and how they felt so that they can clearly identify the benefits of this approach and move towards becoming more accustomed to kindness. Empowerment results through taking responsibility for thoughts, feelings and actions from this moment forth, in a kindly way.

Having developed more resilience and the capacity to have a go at making small changes, perhaps in the way that the client talks to themselves about themselves, or how they relate to others, the inquiry process can explore how this feels.

Compassion can sometimes be used as a subtle form of resistance. For example, a client might say, "I feel so bad about everything, so I'll give myself compassion." This is not what I'm saying here; compassion is deeper than this in that the invitation is to open with a kindly attitude to the full experience, which often actually highlights the lack of self-compassion in any given moment. It really is about developing the capacity to meet oneself right in this moment – a pure act of self-compassion.

As clients begin to feel more confident, it may be that the teacher assists them in finding phrases that they can say to themselves as they become more attuned to their inner wise and compassionate voice. Examples of phrases are:

May I be happy (insert their name).
May I be healthy (insert their name).
May I be peaceful (insert their name).
May I live my life with ease and with kindness (insert their name).

Inquiring into the effects of the personal phrase that they have created for themselves can be revealing. Again, there's a sense of "doing" something to help alleviate suffering and promote their own wellbeing.

During this process, the teacher can highlight the possibilities and changes that begin to become more evident in the client's relationships with others. I have always thought of myself as a kind and compassionate person, having looked after family members during my childhood, becoming a nurse in my late teens, and taking on roles, subconsciously, that meant I looked after others. It was only when I was diagnosed with cancer in 2013 that I had to fully give myself over to the care of others, entrusting my life to them. My mindfulness practice served me well, but only to a point. It was at this time of desperate vulnerability, not knowing whether I was going to survive the illness, that I discovered the true meaning of self-compassion and self-care. Those who have known me well over the years, through friendships and teaching, said that they noticed a significant shift in the way that I spoke, interacted and "felt" to them when I subsequently delivered practices and guided inquiry. This is because I had become truly authentic, balancing mindfulness and compassion equally and embracing them into my life fully.

EXAMPLES OF QUESTIONS

How can you change what you do to help you nurture yourself more deeply?

Now that self-kindness is becoming more familiar, how can this approach be introduced into other areas of your life?

What does it feel like to know that you have a choice in this situation, from a place of self-kindness?

Which habits do you now think it would be helpful to start to let go of, and what other habits would you like to develop more of to support yourself further?

Do you sense that there are possibilities here that you can take forwards into your relationships with others, enabling you to be kinder to yourself and others at work, within the family, socially or in any other interaction you have with people?

Process 6: Sustainable change

What clients have learnt in their meditation practice (for example, being kind when critical thoughts arise, not being as harsh or judgemental on themselves, noticing the discomfort when they change things, or becoming aware of what they do and how they feel) can now come to the surface, impacting on their lives to create a new and fresh way of being. It is of paramount importance that a client pays attention to these new ways of approaching life, with the clients now bringing mindful awareness to the impact self-compassion and compassion for others are having in forming new and more supportive habits and relationships.

Learning to be more self-compassionate can promote self-acceptance, being OK with things just as they are: the emotional turmoil, the inner critic, warts and all. In this way clients can be taught how to develop strategies to soothe their emotional reactivity and feel more empowered and resourced to deal with the vagaries of life.

Once this change has been explored and nurtured deep within, over time, this more self-compassionate approach can lead to the capacity to maintain positive states, become emotionally resilient and recover more readily from negative states, and be generous internally and externally. It can then percolate to the surface, resulting in joy and happiness for all to see.

Consider this scenario: Sandra commented that as a result of taking part in the mindfulness course she noticed that she was limiting herself about going on public transport, especially trains. She became aware that she was so concerned about what she might do if someone was sitting in her designated, pre-booked seat when she got on the train that she would not sleep well the night before in anxious anticipation of this scenario. Mindfulness helped her to see this relationship, and when she became aware of it she developed skills around how to be compassionate to herself. She had a health condition that necessitated her having to sit down and saw that pre-booking a seat was a way of taking care of herself. She also developed the skills around how to communicate with others in a compassionate and boundaried way. This layer of inquiry helped her see this so clearly; she now noticed her patterns of thought and consequential life-limiting behaviour around travel and had the tools to utilise should that situation arise. She now travels far and wide and her life has opened up profoundly – she visits friends and family and pursues all sorts of interests that were closed to her before. When I asked her several months later whether she had ever had to ask someone to get out of her seat, she said, "I don't remember!" Now that is certainly a dramatic shift over a relatively short period of time.

The teacher can prove to be very supportive during this process too, flagging up the differences they have perceived, perhaps, and inquiring into the effects this approach has had on the client's life. It is where a sense of expansion often arises, whereby the participant touches into the endless possibilities that can manifest in response to this new way of being, of feeling part of a greater whole and recognising the potential for profound change.

Once a client has experienced the power of self-compassion, they can start to practice compassion for others from a place of resourcefulness. Their cup is full and they are able to share with others, knowing that they can top the cup up once more by being self-compassionate whenever the need arises. This has the potential to engender profound change in their relationships with others: allowing the opportunity for genuine forgiveness, finding abiding calm when those around are agitated or distressed, choosing to create space between themselves and toxic relationships, and making time for enriching relationships to flourish.

Sometimes clients can even become a little evangelical, wanting everyone around them to experience the freeing and substantial changes that they have as a result of practice and inquiry. The excitement is often tangible. The teacher can steady the ship a little, explaining how others might not be ready for this and that we cannot force change in others – even though they may be in awe of the changes they observe, they have to actively want this for themselves. This is where mindfulness helps in becoming more grounded and seeing things in perspective once more.

Compassion leads to the capacity to maintain more positive states and recover more readily from negative ones. It cultivates generosity and focus as a response to reduce mind-wandering. As we go around and around the cycle, we start to develop a deepening awareness, compassion and appreciation of suffering. This helps us to feel into the connection with the rest of humanity.

EXAMPLES OF QUESTIONS

Can we take a little time reflecting back on what you have learnt and the changes you have made to nurture yourself more deeply?

Now that you have brought more kindness to your practice and life, can you see how else you can apply these skills to create more change?

Has anyone else in your family noticed the changes in you and, if so, what have they said?

What are you going to do now to support yourself more fully?

What are you aware that you need right now to support yourself at this time of change?

Now that you are aware of the benefits of bringing kindness into this situation, perhaps you might be more confident in bringing it in elsewhere when you notice an opportunity. Do you think this might be a possibility for you?

This, of course, is by no means the end of the story – it never is, which is why I have developed a model that is cyclical in nature. With recognition of the changes, a client can become acutely aware of many other aspects of themselves that may need some attention and kindness, and the cycle begins again.

The teacher can facilitate a client in seeing a destructive pattern of behaviour and teach them compassionate ways of managing it with ease and kindness. However, this can often be just the beginning in that the more they realise one pattern, the more they start to identify others. This presents further appreciation of additional opportunities available to bring kindness to themselves at every level, to focus and avoid mind-wandering, and to connect on a deeper level with themselves and humanity...so the virtuous cycle continues!

Inter-relationships

You will see from the model that there is a flow between these stages and processes, with each stage laying foundations for the next. One thereby develops a deeper self-understanding and learns new ways of dealing with difficulties and how to be kinder to oneself and others, both on the surface and from deep within.

Although the arrows go clockwise, life is never this straightforward and there will be times when a teacher will need to change direction or move forwards or backwards. This is only natural and to be expected. Sometimes it's helpful to linger longer in a particular stage to ensure that they become too familiar and embedded and don't feel too rushed.

There are also links between different processes across the cycle: a link between processes 1 and 6 arises from the development of increased awareness of mindfulness in the first instance and how it feels to fully embed mindfulness into life, with an attitude of compassion. Processes 2 and 5 are linked as one reflects upon what happens when one starts to become mindfully aware, and what happens to this awareness as it becomes imbued with kindness. Finally, processes 3 and 4 are linked through the exploration of how what one discovers through mindfulness can be balanced and begin to stimulate wise action in a warm and more wholesome way.

There are no timescales here and no "ideal" as we're all beautifully unique human beings. Thus, a good teacher will pace a client as they gracefully walk, side by side, around this cycle.

Chapter 3

EXPLORING THE NEUROSCIENCE OF MINDFULNESS AND COMPASSION

Dr Trudi Edginton

It is clear that embedding mindfulness and compassion practices into everyday life creates a wealth of opportunities for authentic personal change that are accompanied by significant, measurable effects on psychological wellbeing, physiological health and neurobiological function.

Within our teaching it can be incredibly helpful to provide some information about the neurobiological mechanisms in the brain that underpin these changes and also to introduce some neuroscientific principles to your clients.

This is often a perfect opportunity to notice what comes up for you as you contemplate teaching neuroscience! For some of you it may feel completely natural, or dare I say even quite exciting, but for others it can be quite daunting. I know that for me it was the scientific evidence that piqued my interest in mindfulness and compassion, but I am conscious that I have a background in cognitive neuroscience and felt very comfortable and fascinated by everything that is neuroscience. I am also sufficiently confident to admit that even expert neuroscientists don't know everything about the brain and that it is truly OK to say that you don't know the answer to a particularly difficult question about the brain. I am always so impressed by the brilliant and challenging questions that I get asked about neurons and chemicals in the brain and how they link to our thoughts, memories, emotions and behaviour, and I enjoy sharing the truly authentic wonder at the remarkable processes that are happening in our brain – right now! As I am thinking, typing and sharing my thoughts that have been generated in my mind, you will be reading, thinking and making new connections in your own brain! Our brain is the only organ in the body that we use to study its own workings and mysteries and to contemplate our thoughts and feelings with equanimity and kindness.

Introducing neuroscience

In this chapter I will outline some of the techniques that I use in my teaching to introduce neuroscience in an engaging and meaningful way. I always find it helpful to use metaphors, hand-drawn images (which can also offer some light-hearted relief and valuable teaching points about the lack of perfection or resemblance to the object in mind!) and personal stories to bring the material to life with passion and enthusiasm. All of these can be adapted to become meaningful to you in order for you to feel that you are coming from an authentic place.

Within my teaching I think it is really important to link neuroscience to our felt sense of the world, towards the experiential and "heartfulness" parts of our being, to resonate and truly augment our connection with our inner selves and each other.

Before embedding neuroscience into your teaching, it can be incredibly helpful to familiarise yourself with some of the pervasive neuromyths that often come up as questions or in discussions. These myths are so entrenched into certain settings that even some neuroscience students and educators find it difficult to differentiate between fact and fiction. We can be confident that it is not true that we only use 10 per cent of our brain, or that children are either left brain or right brain learners or that the internet is damaging our brains or causing autism or that brain training products can prevent cognitive decline more than other social or cognitive activities. For a lively, expert and thoughtful account of the promulgation of these myths I would highly recommend Christian Jarrett's (2014) book *Great Myths of the Brain*, where he also identifies the roots of these myths and discusses why they are so compelling.

As a cognitive neuroscientist and mindfulness teacher I am truly fascinated by the powerful effects of mindfulness and compassion that are seen in the brain, body and mind. We know that these practices offer a gentle but effective way to still the mind and connect with our inner selves with kindness, and without judgement, to relieve stress, tension, pain and discomfort and to regulate our mood, emotional reactivity and difficult thoughts.

Attentional mechanisms

Often the focus of our inner experience is determined by the attentional spotlight that we either carefully place there or that can be pulled towards other material without our conscious intention. Using a spotlight metaphor for attentional processing is a perfect example of a beneficial metaphor that is firmly rooted in the neuroscience and cognitive theories of attention. The analogy allows us to explain how we can magnify our focus on something narrow and specific or widen our attentional gaze. Our attention can sometimes be divided or easily distracted – we have a Supervisory Attentional System (Norman & Shallice 1980) that allows us to function effectively on autopilot until something novel or important overrides the automatic attentional processes. The example of driving a car is particularly useful here: the novice is overwhelmed by the multiple elements of driving a car and responding to the environment whereas the expert can drive for miles without being consciously aware of their familiar route/journey. It can be quite reassuring for people if you explain that they are not the only ones who have had this somewhat disconcerting type of experience, and that these shortcuts reflect the brain's attempt to be efficient and are linked to the lack of attention that we all experience at times.

Immersive mindfulness and compassion techniques and inquiry can help us develop a greater sense of awareness and understanding of these automatic processes. Bringing our awareness to these attentional shortcuts can provide us with more opportunities to fully engage with our moment-to-moment experiences. Deepening our practice and inquiry can help us find ways to gently but intentionally direct our attention by enhancing attentional control and flexibility.

We can also highlight the characteristics of our attentional systems, that is, we become easily distracted or captured by negative thoughts or worries about the future, which are, by their very nature, compelling and incredibly difficult to disengage from. There is a very good reason for this, which I often share in my teaching to facilitate self-compassion and self-awareness, and it makes perfect sense when we consider the evolutionary design of the brain as a fundamental teaching point for mindfulness and compassionate inquiry.

Evolution of our brains for threat detection

Essentially our brains have been designed to detect any threats that may be viewed as a potential risk to our safety. From an evolutionary perspective we can easily see the advantage of being able to respond and react quickly to danger. It is no surprise that this powerful detection system is the oldest part of the brain and is often referred to as the "reptilian brain" to reflect its evolutionary age. Across the animal kingdom this system is managed by the left and right amygdalae, two small, almond-shaped structures that can be found deep within each hemisphere of the brain. The amygdalae are highly reactive and rapidly respond to external threats with the co-ordinated release of adrenaline and cortisol to prepare the mind, body and brain for action. Typically, the mind is drawn towards the most salient or significant information, the body will be mobilised in anticipation for a flight, fight or freeze response and some regions of the brain will be temporarily shut down whilst other regions are activated.

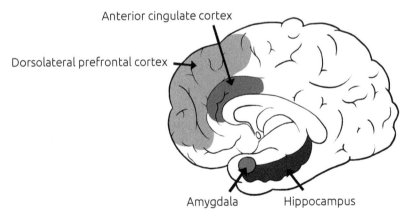

Figure 3.1 The amygdala and hippocampus. The amygdala and the hippocampus work together to detect threat by responding to emotional content in the present by linking to past experiences and emotional memories.

In contrast, the prefrontal cortex is a sophisticated and highly deve-loped "newer" region of the brain that is often likened to the conductor of an orchestra or the CEO of a global company! This part of the brain is responsible for contemplation, detailed analysis, planning, time perception and chronesthesia (most commonly referred to as "mental time travel"). Highlighting our unique mental time travelling skills can resonate deeply and can highlight the bittersweet qualities of our remarkable cognitive abilities. Chronesthesia gives us incredible opportunities to cast our minds back to the past to recall memories of our childhood, friends, special events or holidays. We can also use this ability to contemplate the future and use our imagination to create novel ideas, art and new connections. Unfortunately, this same skill can also lead to the recollection of painful or negative memories, depression and rumination about the past or fear, anxiety and worry about the future.

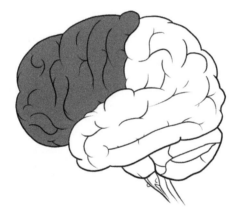

Figure 3.2 The prefrontal cortex. The prefrontal cortex co-ordinates our executive functions, allowing us to plan, focus, make decisions and contemplate the past, future and present.

The distinction between our old reptilian brain and our newer, more sophisticated prefrontal cortex is an aspect of brain development and evolution that we can use to explain a number of our natural instincts, patterns of behaviour and difficulties.

In times of danger or perceived threat the prefrontal cortex region is deactivated by the amygdalae, which means the brain will respond to the threat in a more instinctive way. In the event of being chased by a predator the fact that our thinking (higher) brain is essentially switched off seems somewhat strange; however, this automatic, instinctive mechanism helps us survive the immediate threat and escape potential danger. For some people who have experienced trauma, understanding these mechanisms can be enlightening and therapeutic as they realise that their brains were focused on trying to survive in that moment and so normal sensory awareness, decision-making and behavioural responses were not in their conscious control.

As we are all too aware, modern-day threats are very different to those faced by our ancestors. Thankfully, we don't often get chased by predators on the savannah; instead we are subjected to highly convincing and sustained potential threats to our core selves that hijack our primitive stress response systems. These threats tend to be viewed as very personal, negative and full of intent and they have powerful effects on our psyche. Unfortunately, in these situations, the amygdalae act as Teflon for positivity and magnets for negativity; the negative thoughts and fears can become very compelling and can easily spiral into rumination, worry, low mood and self-doubt.

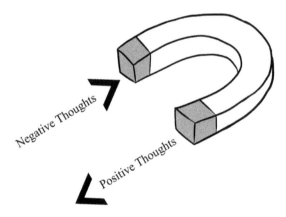

Figure 3.3 Brains attract negativity and repel positivity. Brains have the tendency to be magnetic for negativity but they often deflect positivity.

The sustained nature of these more personal threats can feel overwhelming and the ongoing "battles" that ensue between the old and new brain regions can feel circular, relentless and exhausting – essentially going nowhere.

Highlighting this disparity between the old and the new parts of the brain beautifully demonstrates the mismatch that we face with the complexities and challenges of our modern world. The fact that our brains respond in a dual fashion with both an instinctive and an analytical response means that we are left to manage the confusion that is generated from a range of different threats. This inner conflict can leave us with highly self-critical, negative thoughts and difficult feelings (for example, shame, blame and humiliation) that feel overwhelming, all-consuming and of our own making, which is clearly not the case. Computer hardware and software metaphors are well suited to illustrate these ideas: essentially we have to navigate an increasingly sophisticated modern world with complex cognitive demands whilst running on out-dated software within our brains (Gilbert 2009, p.406). This analogy can be easily expanded to highlight the added frustration in realising that our brains don't have any off-switches or pause buttons to allow us to stop the relentless over-thinking, comparisons, worries and stress, especially when we are alone at night and trying to go to sleep.

Physiological impact of acute and chronic stress

All MBSR and mindfulness and compassion courses focus on the impact of stress, and scientific research has established a strong evidence base for the link between stress and our thoughts, emotions and bodily sensations. In addition, we know that chronic levels of stress influence neurochemical levels and neuronal connections, ultimately changing the volume and the structure of the brain and impacting on our physical health. It is well established that stress contributes to the development of many health conditions such as Irritable Bowel Syndrome (IBS), migraine, skin conditions, alopecia and pain, highlighting the powerful impact of long-term stress. We also know that long-term stress and depression can reduce the volume of certain parts of the brain, especially the left and right hippocampi, regions of the brain that are involved in learning and memory. The hippocampi are part of the limbic system that connects with the amygdalae and surrounding cortices, and these connections underpin the formation of emotional memories and emotionally salient attentional biases.

Exposure to chronic stress over an extended period of time disrupts the levels of the main stress hormone cortisol, which is responsible for the loss of synaptic connections in the frontal cortex and hippocampi. This synaptic loss can be measured and provides compelling evidence for the link between the external stressors and our brain structure. Structural changes in prefrontal cortex dendrites associated with long-term chronic stress can prevent the hypothalamic-pituitary-adrenal (HPA) axis from returning to baseline and these changes can lead to chronic illness, especially cardiovascular or neuro-endocrine conditions.

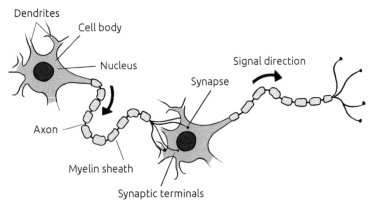

Figure 3.4 Practice increases neuronal connections. Neurons are specialised cells in the brain that are designed to receive and transmit information from dendrites along the axon via electrical impulses and the release of neurotransmitters (chemical messengers). New experiences create new neuronal connections that increase the structure and volume of grey matter in specific brain regions.

Interestingly we can also highlight increases in hippocampus volume that reflect the development of new synaptic connections. A perfect example is the dense hippocampi that are seen in London taxi drivers who have to learn the streets of London (Maguire *et al.* 2000). These examples also demonstrate the plasticity of the brain and offer hope for successful interventions that can target synaptic connections and dendritic growth.

Over time the disruptions to other neurotransmitters can lead to changes in cognitive function and mood. Levels of serotonin (the neurotransmitter that is often referred to as the "happy molecule") can be disrupted, with low levels leading to low mood, attentional biases, distorted perceptions, anxiety and sleep problems. These changes also impact on cognitive function, resulting in executive function, memory and concentration difficulties that are all vulnerable to stress and anxiety.

We are all familiar with the impact of anxiety on our performance, whether it's for an interview, driving test or exam, social gathering or public speaking (the latter has been found to be the most stress-inducing activity as it involves public scrutiny, vulnerability and social judgement). For some of us the anxiety can be debilitating and the anticipation or thought of the anxiety can also create even higher levels of anxiety. We then become hypervigilant and do our best to try to avoid anxiety-provoking situations. However, we end up trapped in a perpetual pattern that maintains the anxiety if we use maladaptive strategies such as avoidance, distraction or hedonistic behaviours.

Our sophisticated and faulty brain

Our inquiry can help us notice these temptations, cravings and urges. Understanding the neuronal mechanisms can also help us to "realize that it is not our fault that we have a faulty brain, but it is our responsibility to manage the responses and our future" (Gilbert 2009, p.46).

An explanation of the sophisticated reward system that works to motivate us into action and help us strive for success can be brought into a variety of our practices, whether we are noticing striving, habits, maladaptive behaviours or addictions. We are also highly motivated by hedonistic pleasure and reward, and often use this as a means of making ourselves feel better. However, these rewards tend to be short-lived and highly addictive, such as the pleasurable feelings we get from substances such as sugar, caffeine, nicotine and other recreational drugs and hedonistic behaviours such as shopping, gambling and sex. These behaviours are all mediated by dopamine, a neurotransmitter that is released when we experience pleasure, temptation, craving and physical urges that can be so compelling they can compromise survival.

This is demonstrated perfectly by research that has shown that rats left in a cage in isolation with the choice of water or cocaine will persist in feeding on the cocaine, rather than taking in water. This can sometimes bring up difficult thoughts, memories or fears in the group if people are currently faced with problems associated with addiction in their own lives, so care needs to be taken. It is particularly helpful and poignant to also discuss the follow-up experiments that placed the rats in a stimulating community cage. In this more socially connected and stimulating environment the rats did not choose the cocaine, highlighting the mediating effect of social connection that can activate another influential affiliative drive system in the brain (Alexander, Hadaway & Coambs 1980).

The brain's internal soothing system is activated by physical contact and connectedness. As we feel safe, content and connected, we release a neurotransmitter called oxytocin, which increases our feelings of connectedness, contentedness and safety. In infancy this part of the brain is not sufficiently developed and physical contact, love, warmth and connection are vital for our sense of attachment, safety and ability to self-soothe later in life. Difficulties with self-soothing can lead to insecure attachment, poor emotion regulation and self-criticism, rumination, anxiety and sleep disturbances.

Discussing the impact of sleep disturbances and the challenges associated with falling asleep provides us with another perfect opportunity to highlight the frustrations of having a human brain and to discuss the different roles of the neurotransmitters!

When we are tired and ready to sleep, the brain must shut down certain regions so that the active process of sleep can be initiated to allow the restorative and consolidation processes to begin during the four stages of sleep. However, in order to activate sleep, the brain has to first alter the brain waves to switch from alpha waves, which reflect a busy working mind, to slower, less active, sleep-related delta waves. I am certain that all of us have had the experience when our brains are captured by a particularly compelling thought or worry and we simply can't switch off and go to sleep. The harder we try to sleep, the harder it becomes!

When we fall asleep there is a carefully orchestrated sequence of events that both activates and inhibits certain neurotransmitters. As a result, certain regions in the brain can then be deactivated. This allows the brain to get on with the important task of processing all of the information from the day. While we sleep, the hippocampi, which usually encode all of our new experiences and memories, are disconnected, explaining why most of our dreams remain elusive. Switching off the memory system while we sleep is vital to ensure that we can discriminate between our waking life and the strange phenomena that make up our dreams! Most of our dreams have the strange quality of randomly travelling backwards and forwards in time, as the region in the prefrontal cortex that is associated with time perception is also switched off. Serotonin, one of the neurotransmitters, is released as we sleep, distorting our perception and creating imaginative and strange connections between real and imagined events, people and ideas. In contrast, acetylcholine, another neurotransmitter, is inhibited, switching off the arousal and attentional systems and relaxing our muscles. Meanwhile, gamma-aminobutyric acid (GABA), a natural sedative, is released, relaxing muscles and preventing us from acting out our dreams while we are asleep. In addition, the brain is working hard to consolidate, process and file away all of the information from the day, ready for the next day. There are times when sleep can be disrupted, which can further impact on the brain's ability to function efficiently. In addition to the effects of anxiety, stress, trauma and/or depression, certain centrally acting medications have an effect on the neurotransmitters involved in the sleep process, giving rise to insomnia, nightmares, frequent waking during the night, early morning waking and feeling more sleepy or unrefreshed when we wake up. Understanding the neuronal mechanisms that underpin these difficulties can help us develop techniques and strategies that can promote greater restorative sleep.

Measurable effects of mindfulness and compassion techniques

There are many useful mindfulness and compassion techniques that one can use to focus the mind, with gentle curiosity, on something that is interesting enough but not too stimulating. A body scan practice at night can be a perfect time to ensure that we have time to pay attention to our internal sensations. Bringing awareness to the present moment to fully savour our internal and external sensory experiences also enhances our ability to strengthen our attention focus, control and flexibility, a process akin to training our muscles in the gym. It can also be very helpful for settling the activity within the mind; as we focus on the body with curiosity, our brain waves change and the active process of sleep can be started. A simple cognitive task such as mentally listing foods, countries or people's names alphabetically is another fairly interesting but not too taxing activity that can help to quieten the mind and help to initiate sleep. (There was infinite wisdom in being told to count sheep!) It can also be helpful to encourage people to explore the difficulties that they experience with sleep and to promote mindful inquiry into the nature of their sensations, feelings, thoughts and worries within an agreed, specified, quiet and contemplative time, before preparing to sleep, where they can spend time developing awareness and going towards difficulties with gentle curiosity and compassion.

Developing compassion and self-compassion is demonstrating awareness of universal suffering and feeling motivated to help with kindness. The term "compassion" has Latin origins *cum* (together/ with) and *pati* (suffer).

Mindful compassion and self-compassion are integral elements within most mindfulness interventions that can be cultivated at a deeper level with compassion-focused training. These practices are particularly powerful and require great care from the teacher. The beauty of most mindfulness interventions is that the courses have been carefully designed to prepare the client for the potential impact of compassion with a range of grounding techniques, emotion regulation, attentional control and equanimity. The careful introduction of a lovingkindness practice can demonstrate the power of the techniques by bringing to mind a loved one and wishing them peace, health and love. The practice then extends to a neighbour, a stranger, the local and global community, including a person with whom you may have difficulties, and the self. Each of these directed practices can create a sense of deep, heartfelt connection and an overwhelming sense of intense love that can be accompanied by an overflow of tears reflecting intense joy, fear and happiness.

The inquiry process and the cultivation of compassion have specific effects on regions in the prefrontal cortex and subcortical structures that, as we have discussed, are important in emotion regulation and learning and memory.

When we consider the prefrontal cortex as a large area of the brain that is involved in decision-making, emotion regulation and attention, we are thinking of this in rather general terms. We can also be much more specific by localising more specific regions in this area that are directly linked to particular cognitive processes and functions. We refer to this process as localisation of function. This allows us to differentiate between the two hemispheres and different parts of the prefrontal cortex using anatomical terms to pinpoint the left or right dorsal, medial, ventral, anterior, posterior and lateral prefrontal cortex areas, which relate to the top, middle, bottom, front, back and side of the prefrontal cortex, respectively, and the left and right orbital prefrontal cortices, which are situated above the eye socket.

One of the key areas within the prefrontal cortex that is activated by mindful and compassionate practices is the dorsal lateral prefrontal cortex, an area that responds when we train our attentional spotlight to develop attentional control. Activation of the dorsal lateral prefrontal cortex, the anterior cingulate cortex and the insula is associated with attentional regulation and cognitive flexibility. If we can develop control of our attentional spotlight and respond flexibly, we are able to develop these cognitive processes to help ourselves gain cognitive control and attentional flexibility.

Modulation of the dorsal lateral prefrontal cortex also contributes to reappraisal processes that are integral to emotion regulation. Being able to consider alternative perspectives is key to developing a more balanced appraisal. It can be helpful to share with the participants that we sometimes need to train ourselves to consider a more neutral appraisal of events or, where possible, adopt a more positive perspective. As we begin to establish these alternative perspectives, we can activate the corresponding regions of the brain to support cognitive reappraisal and better mental health. Connections between the dorsal lateral prefrontal cortex and the anterior cingulate cortex can also reduce rumination by regulating attentional processes. The communication between these different regions highlights the link between the cognitive and the emotional processes involved in regulating our thoughts and feelings.

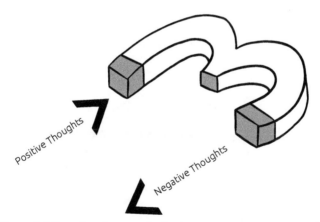

Figure 3.5 Practice changes the brain to attract positivity and repel negativity. Switching the magnet with mindfulness in order to deflect negativity and be more magnetic for positivity.

Developing attentional flexibility and control also recruits the ventromedial prefrontal cortex, the hippocampi and the amygdalae to further develop emotional regulation and control. Bilateral neuronal connections from these prefrontal regions form a dynamic network with the limbic system. In this way the prefrontal cortex can modulate the amygdalae responses to emotional stimuli to soothe and flatten the instinctive emotional responses and regulate the encoding and retrieval of emotional memories that guide our appraisal of emotional experiences.

The medial prefrontal cortex is a central region of the prefrontal cortex that works in tandem with other areas in the brain, including the posterior cingulate cortex, the insula and the temporoparietal junction. The neuronal circuitry and activation between these regions is also responsible for the cognitive shift in self-referential processing that we see following mindfulness- and compassion-based practices. These changes lead to greater levels of empathy and a shift in perspective-taking. We also see the benefits of these changes for the processing of body awareness, facilitating the exploration, curiosity and attunement of bodily sensations that form part of our interoceptive awareness.

In addition, the hippocampi, the auditory cortex in the superior temporal gyrus and the superior colliculus are associated with the binding of multisensory stimuli, bringing a richness to the quality of our experience and our emotional memories. When we ask our clients to pay attention to their internal and external sensations and experiences, we are encouraging them to connect with the multi-sensory nature of everyday experience and to savour the intensity of perception.

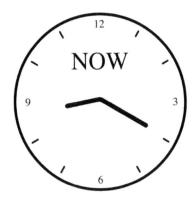

Figure 3.6 Being present in the here and now.

The culmination of all of these new connections gives rise to measurable changes in the brain. At a structural level we can measure changes in neuronal connections between different regions of the brain, and we can measure the thickness of cortical areas by calculating the density of the new synaptic connections. The development of new dendritic connections occurs with the formation of new experiences, new information and the creation of new memories to form the grey matter of the brain.

The evidence for mindfulness-induced changes in the brains of meditators has been supported by a range of neuroscientific studies that have found increased cortical thickness in the left frontal lobe (Lazar *et al.* 2005; Lutz *et al.* 2008), increased grey matter and activation in the hippocampi and decreased volume and activation of the amygdalae (Lazar *et al.* 2005) that reduce their reactivity and/or hypersensitivity.

In addition, studies have been able to measure changes in the anterior and posterior cingulate cortex the insula and the temporo-parietal junction and increased brain connectivity in meditators (Hölzel *et al.* 2011).

There have also been a number of studies that have demonstrated changes in the types of electrical brain waves and changes in the synchrony of brain waves between the two hemispheres in people who have completed mindfulness meditation courses (Lomas *et al.* 2014). These brain waves are detected by placing electroencephalography (EEG) sensors on the scalp that can detect electrical activity in different brain regions. Different brain waves have different electrical frequencies that can be measured and used to determine whether the brain is hyperaroused, focused, contemplative or relaxed. I find it helpful to be able to briefly describe the changes in the different brain waves to explain that beta waves are associated with anxiety and racing thoughts, alpha waves reflect mental focus and concentration, and theta waves are associated with a deep relaxed state and contemplative thinking.

Interestingly, the research findings point to the ability of meditators to be able to pay attention and be focused whilst also being calm and contemplative with an expected pattern of reduced beta waves, increased alpha waves and theta waves. Related studies have also shown changes in Heart Rate Variability that reflect the flexibility of the physiological arousal system. The arousal system needs to be able to respond effectively with increased activation at times of acute stress for action but it also needs to be able to switch to a calmer state of arousal to reduce constant hyperarousal and hypervigilance, which can be detrimental to long-term physical and psychological health. The importance of vagal tone is of particular interest here as the vagal nerve is key to soothing physiological arousal. The vagus nerve is activated with deep, slow breathing, which we all know is a central feature of mindfulness and compassion interventions. As we bring our attentional awareness to the breath and the bodily sensations, we effectively increase vagal tone and control to soothe our nervous system and bring about change.

The synchronicity of mindfulness and compassion practices that bring focus to the breath, the body and the mind, is able bring about long-lasting changes to increase interoceptive awareness, soothe the physiological arousal system, settle our thoughts, and regulate our attentional processes, cognitive appraisal processes, equanimity and emotion responses.

The compassionate mindful inquiry process is key to this process to strengthen the connections between mind, body and brain. Allowing clients to discover the links between their bodily sensations, their thoughts and their feelings is paramount to the experiential nature of mindfulness and compassion. For some clients this may be the first time that they notice that these elements of their humanity are inextricably linked, and this discovery is powerful. Linking their personal exploration of these effects to what we know about the brain and the body can support their understanding of our shared humanity and the cultivation of self-compassion and a compassionate approach to others.

I also find that embedding some neuroscientific principles and explanations in an engaging and accessible manner can be a useful tool to provide scientific evidence and support for the range of techniques and practices that we embody and share with our clients. It is for that reason that we have also incorporated these principles into the Compassionate Mindful Inquiry Neuroscience Model.

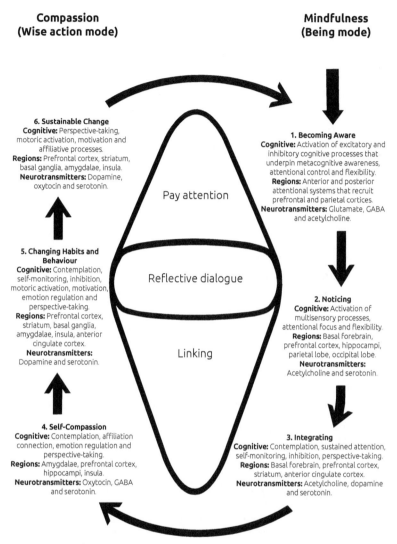

Compassion
(Wise action mode)

Mindfulness
(Being mode)

6. Sustainable Change
Cognitive: Perspective-taking, motoric activation, motivation and affiliative processes.
Regions: Prefrontal cortex, striatum, basal ganglia, amygdalae, insula.
Neurotransmitters: Dopamine, oxytocin and serotonin.

Pay attention

1. Becoming Aware
Cognitive: Activation of excitatory and inhibitory cognitive processes that underpin metacognitive awareness, attentional control and flexibility.
Regions: Anterior and posterior attentional systems that recruit prefrontal and parietal cortices.
Neurotransmitters: Glutamate, GABA and acetylcholine.

5. Changing Habits and Behaviour
Cognitive: Contemplation, self-monitoring, inhibition, motoric activation, motivation, emotion regulation and perspective-taking.
Regions: Prefrontal cortex, striatum, basal ganglia, amygdalae, insula, anterior cingulate cortex.
Neurotransmitters: Dopamine and serotonin.

Reflective dialogue

2. Noticing
Cognitive: Activation of multisensory processes, attentional focus and flexibility.
Regions: Basal forebrain, prefrontal cortex, hippocampi, parietal lobe, occipital lobe.
Neurotransmitters: Acetylcholine and serotonin.

Linking

4. Self-Compassion
Cognitive: Contemplation, affiliation connection, emotion regulation and perspective-taking.
Regions: Amygdalae, prefrontal cortex, hippocampi, insula.
Neurotransmitters: Oxytocin, GABA and serotonin.

3. Integrating
Cognitive: Contemplation, sustained attention, self-monitoring, inhibition, perspective-taking.
Regions: Basal forebrain, prefrontal cortex, striatum, anterior cingulate cortex.
Neurotransmitters: Acetylcholine, dopamine and serotonin.

Figure 3.7 The Compassionate Mindful Inquiry Neuroscience Model.

Compassionate Mindful Inquiry Neuroscience Model
Process 1: Becoming Aware

When we pay attention to our present moment, we see activation of excitatory and inhibitory cognitive processes within the anterior and posterior attentional systems in the brain. These attentional processes are activated or inhibited by the effects of two fast-acting neurotransmitters, glutamate and GABA, which work in combination to maintain a delicate balance that is required to either suppress or attend to information. Our brains need to be able to activate and suppress information and we need to be able to switch between activation and inhibition in order to be cognitively efficient. These processes facilitate our ability to self-monitor and develop metacognitive awareness, the ability to think about our own thinking. The neurotransmitter acetylcholine also plays a key role in the co-ordination of attentional arousal, activation and inhibition. As we age, the levels of acetylcholine naturally decline and we can notice changes in our inhibitory and attentional control and our ability to self-monitor.

Process 2: Noticing what happens

When we direct our attentional focus, we bring intentional attentional processes and rely on attentional flexibility so that we can develop attentional control. We also activate multisensory perceptual binding mechanisms that bring meaning and richness to our internal and external sensations and experiences. Cholinergic projections in the basal forebrain direct acetylcholine to the prefrontal cortex to enhance attentional processes and mediate the multisensory binding processes. The release of serotonin is associated with the perception of sensory and emotional information. These processes integrate information across the parietal lobe, occipital lobe, prefrontal cortex and the hippocampi.

Process 3: Integrating

As we develop more sustained attentional focus, we see the contribution of inhibitory processes that underpin deep contemplation, self-monitoring and perspective-taking. These processes are associated with activation in the prefrontal cortex and the anterior cingulate cortex, which are mediated by the cholinergic system. We also see greater activation in the striatum that is associated with dopamine release, which modulates reward, pleasure and motivation.

Process 4: Self-compassion

As we cultivate deeper levels of contemplation, connection and affiliation, we notice greater emotion regulation, perspective-taking and soothing. These changes are associated with the release of oxytocin, GABA and serotonin, which modulate mood, feelings of connectedness and safety. These neurotransmitters mediate changes in the prefrontal cortex, the insula and the hippocampi and they are known to flatten amygdala reactivity.

Process 5: Changing habits

As we cultivate changes in habitual patterns of behaviour, we see simultaneous changes in contemplation, self-monitoring, emotion regulation and perspective-taking that are linked to changes in motivation. These motoric and motivational changes are associated with the release of serotonin and dopamine that gives rise to changes in mood, habit formation and reward via connections to basal ganglia, amygdalae, insula and the anterior cingulate cortex.

Process 6: Sustainable change

As we establish new patterns of behaviour, we see further changes in contemplation, self-monitoring, emotion regulation and perspective-taking, which become habitual. This wise action fosters compassionate connections with others. These long-lasting changes are associated with the release of oxytocin, serotonin and dopamine that gives rise to changes in affiliation, mood, habitual behaviour and social reward via connections to striatum, amygdalae, insula and the anterior cingulate cortex.

The development of the Compassionate Mindful Inquiry Neuroscience Model has been designed to provide a comprehensive guide to the underlying neuronal, structural, cognitive and emotional processes that emerge and become established via compassionate mindful inquiry. It provides a strong foundation for the development of Compassionate Mindful Training and Inquiry that activates and connects interoceptive awareness, cognitive processes, brain regions and neurotransmitter systems associated with long-term emotion regulation, perspective-taking, attentional control, equanimity and rich connections with the self and others.

Chapter 4

MODELLING A COMPASSIONATE MINDFUL TEACHER

Opening to the connection and interconnectedness that mindfulness brings into your life, with fullness and wholeness, results in a life led with heartfulness, grace and unending joy. Living a congruent life affects all that we say and do, the choices we make from moment to moment, and the relationships we build with other people and this beautiful world in which we live.

Please note that there is an assumption in this chapter that you are either training to teach or are already teaching mindfulness, and I am offering suggestions as to what needs attending to so that you can model a mindful and compassionate teacher.

The essential ingredient

Without question, having one's own regular personal mindfulness practice is absolutely the most important ingredient to becoming a competent and kind teacher. Unlike so many other teacher training programmes, which necessitate increasing cognitive knowledge, teaching mindfulness and leading inquiry in a compassionate way necessitates self-awareness, self-kindness, exploration and self-investigation, as a result of continued practice.

Without practice there is no anchor, no point of reference to guide or, if necessary, provide the courage to be open to not knowing the answer. Whenever I teach, I find myself continuously dropping back into the familiar experiences of my own practice, particularly during the inquiry process. How can one teach with authenticity what one doesn't actually know and feel at this fundamental level? It is imperative for a number of reasons, and clients will know instinctively if the teacher practises what they preach as it assists resonance with one another.

Practice provides a rich, internal knowledge base that no amount of reading or research can replace. Mindfulness is not a technique to be learnt; it's an attitudinal skill to develop and acquire through sustained and regular practice, which is ongoing.

During supervision I often come across teachers who have followed a regulated pathway, learning mindfulness via a recognised programme such as the Mindfulness-Based Stress Reduction course (MBSR). They have practised for the allotted time, gone through teacher training and come out of the other side to find themselves "stuck". They report being bored of practising the same mindfulness practices on their own, and things become somewhat stale in their teaching. Of course, this can happen over time as teachers often need a fresh perspective on their practice – perhaps a skilful nudge to explore things differently, to bring other aspects to the practice and to reinvigorate and deepen their relationship to their practice and themselves. I would always recommend that teachers continue to attend regular teachings that have an element of teacher-led inquiry and remain supported with supervision from a more experienced teacher and practitioner, thereby sustaining growth and development which will be reflected back through their own teaching.

In order to teach others to lean into their own suffering and hold this exploration tenderly, the teacher needs to have done the same, allowing the practice to become the container to permit them to do this fully and effectively. Passionate teachers are those who have fully investigated their own suffering and been supported by their practice to discover new ways of relating to and transmogrifying it.

Whenever I am teaching a group the MBSR programme, I revisit these practices so that I am experiencing them with the clients. I would, therefore, often concur with them when they comment about their experiences, saying for example that I felt the same way during the practice yesterday. Therefore, another benefit of practice is that clients see that there's no trick here – there's no hierarchy in relation to practice with "special" practices for the more competent practitioners. Clients learn that they do not need to and are not expected to aspire to higher, more complex practices, and this comes as a stabilising relief.

Because there is no hierarchy of practice, teachers and clients alike share a common humanity, so there's an understanding that we're all touching and then delicately leaning into our suffering on a daily basis. This really takes any mysticism and sense of striving away from the process, promoting the freedom to share and explore practice experiences on the same level.

The teacher is modelling mindfulness and compassion in the interpersonal space between themselves and their clients. This has the effect of embodying and thus creating intrapersonal skills for the client, often learnt through a process of observation and the feeling tone of the teacher whilst teaching and facilitating inquiry.

The learning process

While learning to drive a car, we learn the skills necessary to be safe on the road but it's only once we've passed our test and are driving without the safety net of dual control and someone else to offer advice, directions and support that we learn the more nuanced skills and gain our confidence and style. Similarly, it takes time and application to become a competent mindfulness teacher who has acquired the necessary skills to lead inquiry and promote exploration and relevance to an individual or within a group setting of any size.

Teaching doesn't all have to be fluent and pre-rehearsed – quite the opposite in fact. And, certainly, sometimes less is more. What I mean by this is that it's sometimes good to discern that it's more appropriate for the client to take a little time to process their own experiences without the teacher digging and delving, poking the stick into the hornet's nest. Going softly, softly is often more supportive, giving time for the client's body, heart and mind to process the insights and changes without the teacher being too assertive and trying to rush the learning to such an extent that it doesn't fully land. When approaching a very timid animal, it's good to take things gently and slowly, making the process feel safe and calm rather than rushing at the creature and scaring it off. So it is too for clients for whom this is a tender process, requiring slow, reassuring compassion and care.

Some clients, quite understandably, simply don't have the resources to play with the edge of their comfort and discomfort, so pushing them too hard and too quickly could exacerbate their distress.

Pacing teaching is important and is easier to achieve when working with an individual rather than a whole group.

Teachers need to stay alive to whether they are trying to satisfy their own needs in the way they are delivering teaching and leading inquiry, maintaining their own interest whilst subsuming the needs of the client.

The four stages of competence

I think it's helpful to reflect on the stages of competence and explore how competence develops and changes over time through the acquisition of cognitive skills and putting these into practice time and again experientially. If you are a mindfulness teacher, perhaps spend some moments asking yourself, "How competent do I feel when faced with a room full of clients starting a course?" Or perhaps further into the programme as they develop their skills, ask yourself, "Am I competent enough to play with their edge of comfort and expand their learning further?" Which cup represents how you feel right now?

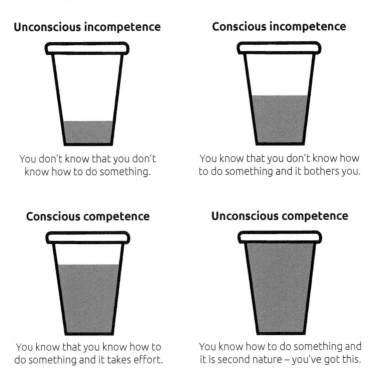

Unconscious incompetence

You don't know that you don't know how to do something.

Conscious incompetence

You know that you don't know how to do something and it bothers you.

Conscious competence

You know that you know how to do something and it takes effort.

Unconscious competence

You know how to do something and it is second nature – you've got this.

Figure 4.1 The four stages of competence.

Unconscious incompetence

In the beginning, we don't know what we don't know, so we are unconsciously incompetent. Rather worryingly, some people are teaching mindfulness from this stance, that is, they do not have their own regular practice yet they start to teach others, usually with the best of intentions, without knowing the territory at all. This is a dangerous place to be as mindfulness is not a panacea and there are occasions when it really can do more harm than good.

Conscious incompetence

The scariest place to be is consciously incompetent. Perhaps you are just starting out becoming a student or newly accredited teacher and you are aware that your skills are somewhat limited in this regard. The good news is that this often precipitates action and perhaps it's the reason you bought this book – you have a thirst to find out more and develop your skill set.

Take your time and listen to your instincts and plug any gaps in learning with reading, watching talks, observing skilled teachers in action...and get some supervision! All competent teachers have been in this position and often remember it very well indeed. Notice what arises in you. Is it a sense of shame, thinking that you should be a better teacher? Notice how this (or any other feelings of not being good enough, unprepared or a little off-balance) manifests in your body and practice some self-soothing. We have all been there and the motto "keep it simple" is very helpful. Perhaps reminding yourself of the intentions of the teaching of that session and smiling softly can result in reconnection and a sense of openness once more.

As I write this, I recall that I was extremely competent working one-to-one but when I taught practices in the early days to groups I had to learn a whole new set of skills. I was so eager to demystify meditation and make it accessible, encouraging people to really feel into the practices and their responses, that my inquiry style was very colloquial. The first question would be something along the lines of "Did you get that?" I soon realised that this closed question approach was not good enough and I set about improving my techniques. I continue to hone my skills, having regular supervision, and continue to teach clients and groups, rather than focusing solely on teacher training.

Conscious competence

This is really hard work. We now know what we need to enable us to lead an inquiry in an effective way, but it takes a lot of thought: thoughts about yourself as the teacher, the curriculum, learning objectives, teaching the practices and other elements of each session, timing, equipment, handouts, downloads, and so on, not to mention managing a group or individual and preparing them for home practice and recording what happened in each session.

It's so helpful at this stage to give yourself time to reflect on what went well. Our brains are designed to seek out the negative and this is what will always come to the forefront of the mind. We need to counter this with a fair and balanced assessment of the session, with an equal amount of time spent on what you would like to do again and carry through to the next session or course. Again, a supervisor has a crucial role in identifying aspects of a teacher that they perceive really enhance their teaching. Applying the sandwich model of communication can be helpful at this stage: exploring what went well, then what could be improved and finishing with another positive aspect of teaching.

At this stage teachers will start to feel very confident in some areas of the course, perhaps when teaching the practices or how they relate to participants. Flagging this up is good practice, helping to bring it to the conscious mind and embed it.

Returning to the new driver analogy, slowly the driver no longer has to think about how to drive; they just jump in their car and go, reaching the final stage of competency.

Unconscious competence

You're there!! You know the course, have experience of working with a whole range of clients, have deepened into the inquiry process and really started to enjoy this privileged and rewarding work. Don't rest on your laurels though; there's always more to learn and one needs to keep the teaching fresh and invigorating, which necessitates energy and prevents a teacher from becoming stale and getting into a rut. Conferences and workshops are great for meeting and listening to a variety of teachers and their own interpretations of the same material. I have learnt so much from these events and would encourage any teacher to keep going to them on a regular basis.

Teaching with integrity and authenticity

These words feel so important to me in my teaching, and becoming my authentic self has arisen from my own practice whilst experiencing the whole gamut of life's ups and downs. Being authentic with myself and the course I am teaching is of paramount importance. It is often so tempting to digress, to be coerced almost into talking about another intervention or being led by a client down a fascinating path of conversation. A teacher needs to remain flexible during the process of inquiry, but it is also important to remain true to what mindfulness is, constantly coming back to the core features and practice with inquiry, over and over again.

Teaching in this way leads to the integrity of yourself and the course, knowing wholeheartedly that what you are doing and the way you are doing it feels absolutely right on all levels. This will go a long way to sustaining engagement and building the trust of the clients during each part of the course or programme.

Embodying compassionate mindful inquiry

So much of our learning comes from non-verbal cues. I'm sure you have experienced being in a room when someone else comes into it and you feel quite different, perhaps uplifted or drained, without knowing specifically why.

Teaching mindfulness begins with the teacher. It is of utmost importance that a mindfulness teacher demonstrates what it looks and feels like to be mindful, by having a mindful presence. First impressions can be very powerful, so the teacher must consider what their clients will see when they meet them for the first time. Is the teacher flustered, unprepared, preoccupied, or at ease, friendly and welcoming?

At the beginning it is inevitable that the teacher will begin teaching from their head, thinking about the practices, timings, information about housekeeping, the model of inquiry, and so on. From the very beginning, though, it's important to take on board that embodying mindfulness is not just about the body but also the mind and the heart.

Keeping a sense of open-heartedness, even vulnerability, is an important aspect of teaching. The tone of inquiry can be varied according to the needs of the client or group and depending on where they are in the process.

It's imperative that the teacher remains compassionate at all times, but there are two types of compassion, both of which have a valuable place in supporting clients:

Tender, gentle, soothing compassion

The teacher can bring a softness to inquiry, moving tenderly through the process with the client, using gentle questions and facilitating a place of easeful safety. This instils a sense of self-acceptance, warmth and comfort.

Embodying self-compassion is important here too, ensuring the teacher has water, is kind to themselves if they forget something and refers to themselves in a kindly manner. I clearly remember being on a Mindful Self-Compassion course with Kristy Arbon.[1] She had a cold and was a bit forgetful and vague in one session. Instead of becoming self-deprecating she just stroked her head and said, "Poor Kristy, you're not feeling too well today are you? There, there." It made more of an impact on me than anything else she taught in that session.

Fierce compassion

This is a compassionate inquiry that helps to develop a client's courageous heart. It may well be that the teacher feels the time is right for a client or group to work with the firmer, stronger side of compassion, instilling a sense of "I've got this" and that they can actively cope with life's challenges. I'm sure we all have seen or even experienced a mother who has had to tap into her inner lioness to defend her child – perhaps this was you? This type of compassion can help clients to feel more capable and less vulnerable. It supports them to act in ways that may protect themselves from others, helps them to make difficult decisions and gives them the strength to act courageously, feel empowered and contribute to reaching their full potential.

It is helpful to consider the most important aspects of the teacher embodying mindfulness. Participants learn best by "sensing" what a mindfulness presence is, without learning it consciously.

---

1   Personal communication (2017) with Kristy Arbon (mindful and somatic self-compassion teacher).

Self-awareness

Know your own patterns. For me an important part of being very present was watching my own patterns to rescue or create ease. These practices have the capacity to create unease, but whatever arises for ourselves or another, if we sit as teachers with genuine ease ourselves, it will help clients to feel safe and give them permission to take as much time as they need.

Getting to know yourself deeply and then moving yourself out of the way can be of huge benefit. The teacher is there to educate, facilitate learning and support the client, and not for any other purpose.

Therapeutic drift

As professionals, in whatever capacity, we all have our strengths and areas of expertise. If you have been working in a particular way with specific client groups for many years, these ways of working with clients will now have become habituated and there will be a raft of unconscious competencies in all that you do and say. Whilst this is phenomenally helpful in your current role, when guiding inquiry after a mindfulness practice there may well be a tendency to drift around in your comfort zone. Therefore, if you are a therapist, used to exploring thoughts and behaviours emanating from past experiences, this may be your default area of focus during inquiry. Another example is if you are a teacher or coach, the emphasis may be upon how to identify difficulties with the client and teach tools or strategies or give presentations that enable the client to change and move forwards in their lives. Whilst none of these elements is incorrect per se, the emphasis may be somewhat skewed towards your professional orientation.

When teacher training, I recognise, for example, how difficult it can be for yoga teachers and yoga therapists to change their language around inquiry and to remain congruent and rooted in mindfulness. Words and phrases often creep in around energies, encouraging relaxation and the benefits of breath control. Having been a yoga teacher myself for 30 years and still teaching, I set my intention as to whether I'm teaching yoga or mindfulness to the class in front of me. The yoga is certainly mindful and compassionate. However, in yoga classes, during both teaching and inquiry, I also talk of *prana* and *yoga nidra* (rather than "body scan"), strengthening the core and breath retention, phrases that I would never bring into pure mindfulness sessions.

Pause for a moment and ask yourself the following questions:

- What is your current job role and what makes you good at it?
- Identify your areas of strength as these will be your default.
- What are your "go to" behaviours when you feel anxious in your role?
- Does this differ from your role as a mindfulness teacher?
- What do you need to do to ensure that your inquiry remains congruent to mindfulness?
- How does your own practice support you in this?
- Are there any other strategies you could use?
- Do you consciously need to bring more authentic compassion to your teaching?

The teacher must, therefore, spend some time contemplating their own safety nets and explore whether their default mode is appropriate and relevant to teaching mindfulness and compassion to a client, on a moment-by-moment basis.

Being alive to your own suffering

Everyone I have trained and supervised, myself included, has suffered and continues to do so. Mindfulness has gone some way to help manage and alleviate their suffering, leading them to want to support others who are struggling with difficulties by using these practices, skills and tools.

Therefore, maintaining an awareness of yourself at all times is of paramount importance. This means knowing how you are physically, emotionally and psychologically throughout the teaching process and looking after yourself. This is especially true when leading inquiry, as balance, equanimity and openness are essential in creating an environment that is safe for clients to disclose whatever they wish. A greater proportion of your attention should rest on yourself in order to stay present, rather than getting caught up in a vortex of the client's story or inquiry responses.

If you are low in energy, feeling unsettled or whatever, adjust the teaching and inquiry to suit. There is nothing to be gained by pushing yourself to do something you're not comfortable with if you're not feeling resourced to deal with the outcomes. Be kind to yourself, play a recording of a practice rather than guiding it yourself, ask another to co-teach with you, put on a YouTube clip about neuroscience or do whatever you need to do to stay connected to yourself and your clients.

Paying attention to what you, the teacher, need in any moment will help you to stay centred and balanced. Inevitably, clients will push your buttons, whether purposefully or not, and suffering will arise. Recognising that it's there, and then employing mindful self-compassion to help ameliorate it, is vital during teaching. It may well be that you decide to pause and guide a breathing space practice because that's what you need to gather yourself and recalibrate. The clients will never know and everyone will benefit!

Being aware when your own suffering is triggered is essential, and then knowing how to handle this in the middle of an inquiry process comes from your own practice of mindful breathing, mindful body scan, mindful grounding and self-soothing. Having established and familiar resources will enable you to deal with any difficulties that arise and is crucial when teaching this open-hearted work.

In his book *Anger: Buddhist Wisdom for Cooling the Flames*, Thich Nhat Hanh (2001) uses the analogy of being a firefighter when describing the importance of therapists looking after themselves when they, too, may well be in the zone of fire. He explains that we must have our own equipment to deal with difficulties arising within us, igniting reactivity, sparked off by something a client does or says.

This equipment comes in the form of awareness through our own practices and knowing ourselves, our own "hot buttons"; then, knowing how to handle the rising heat through self-care and wisdom so that we can bring our own temperature back down so that the client–teacher interaction is not disturbed or affected unduly.

That said, speaking from a place of truth and knowing will resonate more with a client than clever words or carefully planned phrases. The client will "feel" it and know that you are connecting with their suffering. Stay alert, though, by using a beginner's mind, with an awareness that the client does not have your resources and has not yet been through the processes that you have. Remembering what it was like for you when you first opened up to your own suffering keeps the teaching content and pace appropriate for the client. Recall times when that sharp beam of awareness of suffering brought you such clarity, like a search light, but perhaps it was also harsh and unforgiving. Your compassion softens the beam, for you and the client, creating warmth and a gentle awareness that creates a sense of being able to cope with whatever is being seen for the first time.

Much of the time it's really important to get the "self" out of the way. By this I mean judgements, reactions, needs, impulses and urges, as well as trying to give your own views or examples too much. Sure, it's helpful to occasionally use stories from your own life to demonstrate how mindfulness can be used in a variety of situations, but this can certainly be overdone.

Through maintaining awareness of our own responses during the inquiry process, we manage to look after ourselves moment by moment and thus our own suffering does not impinge on that of others and the support we give remains impartial and equanimous.

To give an example, Tammy was really very competitive and defensive with me. If I was in the process of teaching, she would often interject, giving an additional fact, always wanting to have the final say. Equally, if something came up that she hadn't experienced, she put up a smoke screen, deflecting the inquiry down a more familiar path or explaining that she had decided to do it differently.

One day, the group were invited to choose an activity to do mindfully at home. They all worked together and agreed to do the same thing so they could support each other between practices. I don't usually teach in this way but they were very keen, so the task was agreed. Unfortunately, it was apparent at the next session that Tammy had forgotten to do this particular activity mindfully during the intervening week so, instead of explaining this, she made up all sorts of excuses and stories, saying she had spent her time on much more important tasks, and was rather dismissive of all those who had remembered and were sharing their experiences.

I have absolutely no issue with anyone forgetting something, but my buttons are pressed very firmly when stories are fabricated and, in doing so, demean others. All I had in that instant was my practice – awareness that my buttons were being pressed, anchoring my attention on my breath and feeling present in my body. I chose to practice deep, compassionate listening, not interjecting, feeding or validating her stories in any way. I was acutely aware that if I spoke there might be an edge to my voice, something in my delivery that felt less than congruent, so I remained still and strong. It helped to defuse the situation and it was clear as she spoke that something clicked in her, a realisation perhaps that I really didn't mind whether she practised or not; it was her choice and her habitual patterns of defence were not related to me but something she needed to attend to for herself.

On reflection, this approach was a combination of tender and fierce compassion. Staying quiet served to give me the opportunity to self-soothe, not feed her flames, protect the others in the group and create space for her to explore what was going on for her and find her own resolution.

Room dynamics and posture

The postural relationship between the teacher and client and/or group has a significant impact on the process of inquiry, and the comfort of and effect upon the teacher is of equal importance to that of the client(s).

Consider the position of the chairs. I would not have chairs facing each other directly when doing this work one-to-one – it's too confrontational and can feel intimidating. It's much better to have them slightly off-centre so there is the opportunity for the teacher and client to feel they can naturally look away, think or pause, rather than constantly making eye contact.

If a teacher is able to adopt a circle or oval, they should consider where they sit within it and the practicalities associated with that in relation to the flipchart, projector, readings, notes and so on.

Also, when conducting inquiry, it might be a little awkward turning directly to the person next to the teacher's side in a tight circle. I like to create a little space around me and sit in a place to ensure that no one is straining their neck but everyone feels included and part of the group.

The teacher also needs to:

• Sit upright – open and receptive.

• Keep their feet on the floor, not tucked up underneath on a chair. It is necessary to stay grounded because the teacher has no idea what will arise during the inquiry process and this helps them to stay prepared.

- Release any physical tension.

- Keep a drink close by – there's often a lot of talking in these sessions.

- Check in to ensure breathing is gentle and rhythmic.

- Remain attentive with good eye contact.

- Demonstrate good listening skills.

- Stay alert, applying the attitudes of mindfulness.

- Be clear when offering teaching, presenting or giving feedback during inquiry.

Developing skills to use the body to elicit responses during inquiry is a useful technique to acquire. For example, leaning towards a client who may be reticent to speak, thereby creating more of a bubble in which they may feel more confident to speak up. Alternatively, if a client is over-sharing, turning away from them a little, perhaps with the shoulder, may halt their flow.

Facial expressions are super important and a teacher's awareness of their quirks and responses can prevent clients feeling ill at ease. Maintaining a sensitive and gentle expression invites inquiry, rather than an overly concerned look, which may be somewhat sycophantic and inauthentic, thereby closing down dialogue.

Using comforting and compassionate gestures (for example, inviting clients to place their hand on their belly) can promote a sense of connection and resonance with them. It might be that you guide clients to do this as part of the practice and then inquire about the changing sensations resulting from introducing and then letting go of this gesture; or you may place your hand on your heart during inquiry as you resonate with what the client is expressing.

Habitual language

As a teacher, you must be acutely aware of the impact of your habitual language used when delivering mindfulness and guiding inquiry.

It's helpful to consider the words you generally use in your daily life, both at work and at home. What are your common phrases and what sense do they manifest? For example, you may be extremely positive in your approach and feel a real sense of passion and desire to teach mindfulness to others, so you may even err on the side of being evangelical. Whilst enthusiasm is great, it sometimes can feel a little overwhelming and the pace too fast.

We all learn in different ways at different speeds and it's possible that swept along by your own energy and dynamism you may try to hurry clients' learning. Your language may reflect this, urging them to keep moving forwards with their learning. These skills can sometimes take time to learn and become embedded, so a beginner's mind is extremely important in this context.

Maintaining your own awareness of thoughts and being attuned to the impact of the resultant words is important: learning to think before speaking. This is yet another reason why it's imperative that you take a thorough assessment and have some sense of each client, as you may need to modify your language in some way to enable clients to understand you fully.

This is not to say that you dumb things down or become bland in style, content and delivery; rather, take note and assess the responses to your inquiry questions, or lack of them. It may be that you need to phrase things in a more client-centred way.

Maintain an awareness of your use of abbreviations and your work-based language if teaching outside of this setting. All professions have their own shortcuts, I know, I have worked in the field of healthcare for the last 35 years and sometimes feel like a fish out of water in other workplace contexts. Be curious – is there a tendency to fall back to this as a default?

Tone and volume of voice

When leading inquiry it is important to be aware of your tone. In an ideal world, you may already have a naturally soothing and gentle voice which lends itself to guiding meditations. This, however, can also have its downsides as the client may be soothed too fully and feel they are being lulled into a state of relaxation. I am sometimes told this by my clients about my own voice, so I try to sharpen my tone and bring clarity of instruction to maintain awareness and attention.

Two students come to mind as I write this. One was a hypno-therapist who had to work hard to move away from the lulling, literally hypnotising voice, tone, rhythm and syntax, to lift it up and put some energy into it. This was especially important during inquiry as this requires investigation and curiosity, not sleepiness and dullness.

The other was an actor who was so used to projecting his voice to the back of a large theatre that each practice he taught was more of a performance than an interaction. His inquiry was more like an act from one of Shakespeare's plays, with emphasis and an over-exaggerated inquisition. Eventually I encouraged him to "act" as if he were a meditation teacher and this did the trick! I taught him to "fake it till you make it" and he became a wonderful teacher.

The tone we use should be the same as our normal speaking voice, not particularly slowed down or put on in any way, as some people do when talking on the phone or in certain situations. This teaches clients that they do not have to have "special conditions" in order to meditate or inquire into their experiences. It helps them to "normalise" the whole process, making it accessible and commonplace in their lives.

The emotional tone is kind and compassionate. Sometimes a soft, tender tone is appropriate, whereas at other times using a stronger compassionate tone may elicit a feeling of strength and a building of resources, leading to the client's motivation to act or perhaps play with the edge of their discomfort more readily, for their own good or that of others.

Naturally it is also important to determine whether a client is hard of hearing and raise your volume appropriately. If there is a person within the group whose hearing is impaired, ensure they are nearest to you or the recording being played, and ask others to turn and look at that person when making a comment, so they can lip read if necessary and maybe increase the volume if that helps. A hearing loop system may also be of benefit.

Pace of the process

The pace of the inquiry process dialogue is important too. Often one of two things will happen. Particularly at the beginning, there may be long silences after you've asked clients to share their experiences. This can feel so awkward, especially if you're a silence-filler. Allow these periods of silence, as usually there's a lot going on in them for clients. They're often exploring their processes after practice, then trying to find the words to articulate what happened, how they felt, what they observed. Of course, if the silence isn't broken after a period of time, it's a good idea to ask a more specific question such as "Did anyone notice a change in temperature in the hands, feet or any other part of the body?" It's an easy question to answer and often gets the ball rolling.

The other and opposite scenario is that one or more clients may have experienced so much during a practice that everything starts to be fed back quite quickly and it's easy to be drawn into their excitable spin and take the inquiry too fast. This might mean that you're skimming too lightly and quickly and not giving enough time for experiences to become embedded, cogitated and flagged up.

At the start of teaching, you too may be a little nervous, which might mean you go a little too quickly, attempting to squeeze everything into the session. Notice this and change posture, deepen the voice, slow down your breathing, ground yourself, have a sip of water or guide a movement practice – whatever it takes to slow you down a bit.

If someone has had a really significant experience – perhaps an awareness that what they identified within the meditation is their habit in real life – I will sometimes pause the group, perhaps even raising my hand a little, before anyone else can jump in and begin feeding back about their experience too. Sometimes feedback can be so profound that I can feel it as well, so I might put my hand to my chest and say something like, "That feels like such a shift for you." Light bulb moments need attention and are to be savoured.

The whole of the group will start to naturally find their own pace. Some groups go fast, particularly those led within a workplace setting. This might be the culture: everyone knows each other well and they already have strong communication channels; or they're emotionally intelligent and a supervision model where inquiry is key to their work (as in social work) is a familiar process. Other groups can perambulate gently along, with space and time aplenty. It's important to know your own responses to these presentations, be good at time management and maintain a balance, perhaps picking up the pace if it's too sedentary, or slowing things down if too speedy.

Linger longer

As my career unfolds, I am noticing how important it is to encourage clients, students and supervisees to linger longer. Processing information takes time, and, for many, this is foreign territory in which they encounter barriers and walls. In my own practice I have noticed how jarring it can be to become aware of thoughts, for example, and then redirect my attention back to the object. It feels quite judgemental and I now linger longer with an experience and watch what happens to the thought when I give it space and attention. As a consequence, I now teach this to clients to good effect.

Similarly, I take a little more time over reading poems, sometimes repeating pertinent lines, or pausing afterwards to let their message or tone linger in the air and land with a feather-like quality. No rushing, no striving, no judgement...just spacious lingering.

Skilful guidance

However glorious this sounds, you will constantly be shifting in and out of doing and being modes of mind, making decisions or choices as to what to do next. When conducting inquiry, being with direct experiences needs to be counterbalanced with teaching points related to the learning objectives of the session, ensuring that clients are developing an understanding of the concepts of mindfulness and how self-compassion enhances their experiences.

You will usually have a guide, plan or course curriculum to follow; you will perhaps be discussing the research evidence or neuroscience relating to the practice but at the same time be trying to hold an open, friendly space for discussions, questions and concepts to bubble up.

Paradoxically you may have been commissioned to address a specific issue in the workplace or with specialist groups and yet you're also letting go of agendas and goal-setting and promoting a sense of non-striving, even though it may be that the course outcomes are being measured.

Interactions within groups

The levels of interaction change and develop during the course process as understanding, appreciation, familiarity with the concepts and each other and their relationships develop.

I often think that the beginning of the course is quite hard work as the group has lots to learn, anxieties arise and thinking is prevalent. There is such a lot of information to impart and a sense of getting everyone up to speed with what mindfulness actually is, what it means to meditate and how to begin utilising these rediscovered skills and new tools in daily life.

One only has to consider Bruce Tuckman's (1965) model, which theorises that teams go through the stages of forming, storming, norming and conforming, later with the addition of adjourning, through time. Although workplace-based, it reflects my professional experience with some groups and is helpful to bear in mind during the teaching process. Of note here is that the storming phase often coincides with the neurological changes in the middle of the course, where there is sometimes a resistance to practice, collusion between clients, and challenges directed towards the teacher as well as the efficacy of the course. These phases are natural stages of the learning and development process for some groups but not all. Knowing about them depersonalises events for the teacher, though they still need addressing.

Participants will be spending some time observing, often subconsciously, what the teacher does or says in response to a range of comments during the inquiry process. Often if a participant has found the practice boring or distressing, they'll apologise to the teacher as they have a preconceived notion that the teacher wants everyone to relish the whole course from beginning to end. This is not what actually happens at all. When a teacher does not seem perturbed by anything that is fed back, this instils confidence in participants to say what they are truly experiencing and leads to trust and honesty for the whole group.

Trust within relationships build and clients reveal more to themselves and others when the teacher resonates with each client individually and the group as a whole. Empathy, compassion and sympathetic joy are essential ingredients in this, giving clients support to open up further and investigate more deeply.

It may well be that this is the first time that they have attended an educational course since school and there are deeply ingrained habits and beliefs around the teacher–student interaction, such as their answers having to be right or pleasing.

I recall one participant, Fiona, who constantly put her hand up when she felt she wanted to contribute to the conversation in some way. This habit was so strong in her that even when I looked at her and asked a question directly, she still raised her hand. I expect there was a lot going on for her at a deeper level around the teacher–student relationship.

It often feels that there is a gearshift in the middle of teaching a course, which comes about for several reasons. Hopefully, people feel less anxious about the course, expectations and with each other; they have started meditating, so their brains will be beginning to change; and they have climbed the steepest part of the new learning curve and have settled into the rhythm of the programme.

This is the point at which teaching becomes more bespoke, really listening to how participants have started to incorporate mindfulness into their lives, with the teacher giving encouraging support to develop these findings that lead to further action and change. This is where I sense in myself a feeling of relaxation and flow. I no longer need to be teaching so much about what mindfulness is but am able to sit back and let the clients tell me how they are interpreting the teaching in creative and effective ways in their own lives.

Communication skills

How a teacher communicates with clients during inquiry impacts significantly on their experience of the process, their learning and development. In Chapter 5 we explore the impact of language, but there is so much more to communicating than simply the words used.

Our styles of communication arise from cultural conditioning, and the teacher will have their own habits of thinking and speaking. Communicating authentically is important. When training teachers I always encourage my students to find their own voice. I don't want them to become mini-mes but to find their own style and phrases that sit well with them.

Marshall Rosenberg (2003) explores how human behaviour stems from attempts to meet universal human needs, and conflict arises when strategies for meeting these needs clash. This inability to meet needs on an individual and societal level is often what initiates an interest in mindfulness for clients.

His proposal is that in order to communicate well we must be self-empathic, connecting with our own needs by noticing feelings, thoughts and judgements as a teacher, without blame. Secondly, he describes receiving what another is saying empathically, with the whole being. As a teacher we can focus on listening for the underlying observations, feelings, needs and requests of the client. Lastly, encouraging a client to express their experiences honestly can lead to them going deeper, touching into what they really need to understand and progress.

So, the needs of the teacher should be given credence, allowing their natural kindness and curiosity to flow into the interactions, supporting the experience of teaching in a way that feels congruent. This has the effect of looking after the teacher whilst dialoguing with a client, so that when a teacher asks a question, saying, for example, "I'd be interested to hear your experience of that practice", there's a true sense of curiosity that feels genuine, friendly and rewarding for the teacher.

Deep listening is key. I strongly believe that much of the power of the inquiry process comes from the capacity of the teacher to listen well, giving the client what is often a unique experience for them: of being listened to on purpose, in the present moment without judgement. At this moment of deep, compassionate listening, the teacher must stop doing anything else and focus entirely on the client, make good eye contact, listen to what is being said and how, use their whole being, have an awareness of their posture, thoughts and judgements and let go of trying to solve the client's problem. Just being is often enough to engender radical acceptance of experiences, for the client, teacher and/or whole group.

Attitudes of mindfulness

Keeping the attitudes of mindfulness at the heart of inquiry provides a firm foundation from which to guide, develop and open to the full experience of the process. There are a number of universally recognised attitudes to hold in mind when conducting inquiry. The practice of mindfulness is rather like cultivating a garden: it flourishes when certain conditions are present. These attitudes can be enfolded into how the teacher presents themselves and conducts inquiry.

1. Beginner's mind

This quality of awareness sees everything as new and fresh, as if for the first time, with a sense of curiosity. A teacher will hear similar comments over and over again, but what keeps inquiry fresh for them is remaining connected to the client, remembering that the client is experiencing this perhaps for the very first time, enabling the teacher to walk in their client's shoes. The teacher may recall when they started to learn practices and began to perceive things in a different way. Connecting to these early sensations can refresh attention and connection to the client's current experiences and support them in seeing things as they really are in this moment in their lives, so that both the teacher and client benefit from this attitude.

2. Non-judgement

This quality of awareness involves cultivating impartial observation with regard to any experience: not labelling thoughts, feelings or sensations as good or bad, right or wrong, fair or unfair, but simply taking note of thoughts, feelings or sensations in each moment. The teacher must also notice judgements arising, which is inevitable, in their own mind. By acknowledging the internal effects of these harsh, negative judgements through personal experience, the teacher can then let them go as they conduct inquiry, which is essential to remaining an impartial and compassionate observer and facilitator.

3. Acceptance

This is the validation and acknowledgement of things as they are, with no need to try to let go of whatever is present. If the teacher is fully accepting of the version of themselves that shows up in that moment, the client will sense into their loving, authentic presence.

4. Non-striving

Striving can lead to contraction, concentration and focusing on achievement, but with the quality of non-striving there is no grasping, aversion to change, or movement away from whatever arises in the moment. Inquiry is a process and it is often a relief for the teacher to let go of the need to strive to "teach". Their role is to provide a container with the right atmosphere for learning to evolve and resources to build when meeting the suffering of themselves and their clients.

5. Letting go

This attitude is one of non-attachment and it is helpful for a teacher to become aware of their own attachments to teaching (for example, a desire to get the message across, grasping for what the teacher wants from the process or a wish to keep it moving forwards) as this will impact on inquiry. Conversely, if the teacher models compassion, moment by moment, all those in attendance will benefit.

6. Patience

Patience can be viewed as a form of wisdom. A teacher who embodies patience demonstrates that they appreciate that a client's learning must unfold in their own time. The teacher must remain completely open to each moment, accepting it in its fullness, giving time and space for whatever arises.

7. Trust

Trusting the process, the practices and the value of inquiry is an important ingredient, I suspect, in leading mindfulness teachers to want to share this approach with others. How can anyone teach without knowing and feeling first-hand that mindfulness is effective? Research has done much to substantiate the efficacy of mindfulness, thereby demonstrating with empirical evidence that this approach can be trusted to elicit change. However, the important aspect is that the teacher learns to trust their own intuition and experience as to how to inquire into their client's feedback, deciding whether to ask soft, safe questions or challenging questions that lead a client to explore beyond their comfort zone, the area of growth and maturity.

8. Equanimity

This quality of awareness involves balance in all things and ultimately fosters wisdom. Having respect for the client's own inner wisdom has the effect of strengthening their belief in their own capacities to move towards freedom from suffering and increased happiness. The teacher creates a container that allows a deep understanding of the nature of change, how we as humans have a tendency to expend an inordinate amount of energy moving towards things we really want, grasping with focused determination and moving away from things we don't like. Equanimity allows teachers to notice when their thoughts, feelings and behaviour are being driven by attraction and aversion, enabling them to come back to the centre. This is rather akin to how a squash player comes back to the "T" at the centre of the court once they've taken their shot, rather than being left off-centre as the next hit is made by their opponent. Therefore, the teacher demonstrates how to be with change with greater balance, insight and compassion.

9. Self-compassion

Being a self-compassionate teacher is a profoundly important quality to cultivate when guiding inquiry.

On the last day of teacher training in Finland, Hanna Karhu,[2] an MBSR student and occupational therapist, expressed the value of self-compassion beautifully, saying, "I've always known it, but now I own it".

Self-compassion is a profoundly important quality to cultivate when practising and inquiring into experiences. It negates self-blame, guilt and criticism, enabling the teacher and client to open to the full expanse of learning and joy that arises from mindfulness.

Holding these qualities in mind, reflecting upon them and cultivating them as best one can will nourish, support and strengthen practice, learning, teaching and inquiry. These attitudes are, of course, interdependent: each influences the others, and by cultivating one, all are enhanced.

Identifying a teacher's qualities

We are all very individual and, as teachers, bring limitless qualities to the inquiry process. Recognising and exalting these qualities and unique differences is important. This acknowledgement of what a teacher naturally brings builds confidence and helps them to develop their own, authentic style. I always like to ask student teachers what they think their friends and loved ones see in them, what is it that's attractive or endearing that means people want to stay connected to them?

---

2   Personal communication (2019) with Hanna Karhu (occupational therapist and mindfulness teacher).

Perhaps taking time to consider your personal qualities that will augment your teaching would be helpful at this stage. Take a moment to reflect and see what arises, then jot these natural qualities down.

For example, I often hear from my students of their concern that teaching mindfulness is quite heavy, agitating and perhaps distressing for the client. I don't disagree that this is sometimes the case, but the opposite is often true too – it can be hilarious! Creating an environment in which clients can express joy, light-heartedness and humour comes from the ability of the teacher to laugh at themselves and see things in perspective. Indeed, this may be the take-away from teaching: because we are aware, we can get ourselves tied up in knots about things and we can all take ourselves and situations too seriously sometimes – there's such learning here.

Intuition

Trusting the teacher's intuitive processes aids inquiry with a client. Intuition arises from personal meditation practice, knowing oneself intimately, and a compassionate attitude towards oneself, developing interpersonal skills from a place of feeling and sensing rather than a cognitive, thinking process. The quality of intuition arises from the teacher's capacity to be open, empathic, kind, vulnerable, honest, respectful, balanced and wise when in the presence of another.

When guiding inquiry, a new teacher may find it easier to follow the process and questions as described in Chapter 2, sequentially. As skill and familiarisation with the process of inquiry develops, the teacher may begin listening to their intuition, bringing additional benefits to the client via questions in relation to the teacher's "sensing" and "feeling" rather than "thinking".

Intuition lends itself to the development of perception, the ability to draw back and see the full picture. If a client is entrenched in their attachment to their story or experiences, a teacher may use their intuition to assist them is seeing things from a different angle.

Teacher's experience

Consider the clients with whom you are leading inquiry. Do you have some knowledge and training in relation to that specific client group? It's also helpful to identify whether additional skills are required for

COMPASSIONATE MINDFUL INQUIRY IN THERAPEUTIC PRACTICE

a specific group and ensure you get training to plug the gaps so that inquiry is informed and professional. It is advisable not to work with a group that you are unfamiliar with and it is important that you are able to adjust the inquiry to suit the specific needs of the individual. Keeping up-to-date with the most recent research for your clients and shadowing or co-teaching alongside those with more experience will be a valuable experience.

The teacher must consider their own patterns of behaviour and their own mind traps as well as their role as perceived by their clients. It may well be, for example, that because the teacher has been through a teacher training process both they and their clients think they are the eternal expert, knowing all the answers to questions, situations arising and, indeed, life! This is one reason why I think it is so helpful to sit in a circle to teach a group and to share the practice with the client(s) whilst bringing an attitude of humility to the interaction.

Whilst inquiring at the end of a course as to what the main key learning was for the participants, Tanya said she was watching me like a hawk for the whole course and noticed how I sometimes said, "I'm just going to take a moment to pause and gather my thoughts before I answer that question." She reports observing me taking a breath or two before responding and that was what she was going to take away and incorporate into her life. She went on to explain that she thought the teacher would know it all off-pat and would just be teaching information and practices almost by rote; what she learnt from her observations was the power of being present and seeing me look after myself during the teaching process.

This demonstrates the assumptions and judgements that clients bring to the teaching process and that it's often not what is said by a teacher but what is experienced by clients by observing the teacher caring for themselves, moment by moment that shapes the key learning.

Who is looking after the teacher?

As John Donne (1959, p.108) said, "no [wo]man is an island entire of itself". However, I do often hear mindfulness teachers saying that they sometimes feel like a lone wolf, working, teaching and enthusing about mindfulness to clients, but what they would dearly like is a community of teachers to connect with.

The teacher wears so many hats when leading inquiry, including that of an assessor, analyser, communicator, teacher, informer, instructor, connector, guide, supporter, giver and receiver, to name a few. Taking on these roles, plus having to stay connected to oneself, adhering to the curriculum, watching the clock and managing group dynamics, is such a lot to hold, that the teacher must acknowledge that they, too, need support.

This taking care, of course, begins with the teacher's own practice. Are you, the teacher, going to a regular group and is inquiry an integral part of this? Also take a little time to evaluate if you have support from family and friends and how perhaps you could elicit and develop this more or fill in the gaps. Are you able to reach out to like-minded teachers, belong to an alumni group, connect with peers via the internet, co-teach, observe teaching, attend continuing professional development (CPD) days or conferences and retreats, for example?

Supervision

I worked for many years in a clinical setting within an organisation where I got very little supervision and therefore I know how debilitating this can be. Ultimately, as a consequence, I was unable to continue offering my skills as I was experiencing early signs of burnout and decided to hand in my notice before something catastrophic happened. Supervision is, therefore, of utmost importance, enabling those of us doing this unpredictable, heartfelt work to have someone else to talk things through with in confidence, feel supported in all manner of ways, know that someone else has "got your back" and fully sense into the knowledge that you are not alone. Do you have a supervisor who offers you the individual and regular support you need? When someone asks you a question during teaching or guiding inquiry that you are unable to answer, to know that you can say, "That's an interesting question to which I don't know the answer, but I'll take it to my supervisor and come back to you," is supportive, empowering, a great learning experience and very professional.

Good Practice Guidelines for Mindfulness Teachers

The British Association of Mindfulness-Based Approaches (BAMBA) (2019) sets out *Good Practice Guidelines for Mindfulness Teachers* working within a whole range of settings. Whether you are a teacher on the regulated teachers list or not, I would strongly recommend adhering to these guidelines as they have been developed and refined over many years and are underpinned with evidence and integrity.

When a teacher is confident and feels "held" themselves, within their teaching role, they are then able to inquire in a natural, friendly manner without becoming caught up with self-conscious concerns. This is when the magic happens.

Chapter 5

LEADING SKILFUL COMPASSIONATE MINDFUL INQUIRY WITH CLIENTS

Sensing into the thread that links one's own practice, inquiry and choices to live life congruently, whilst guiding others, ensures alignment and resonance with one's inner, core values, flowing with ease into the role of teacher and facilitator, seamlessly.

Integrating teaching, guiding practice and inquiry

Folding the experience of practice into the inquiry is what makes this process so powerful. Conducted without boundaries and borders, the observations made during the practice can be explored, shining a light on the complexities of the body, heart and mind and seeing clearly the impact this has on every aspect of life.

Unfortunately for the new teacher, there are no "stock" answers in response to a client's inquiry feedback, but knowing the benefits and potential difficulties arising for a client when guiding any practice is helpful when facilitating inquiry. These are learnt during any mindfulness teacher training programme, many of which will also have been experienced by the teacher in response to their own personal practice. However, these are simply guidelines, providing some anchor points to the process. The teacher will begin to find that sometimes widening the torch beam, creating space for comments and questions to arise, is appropriate. At other times, a narrow focus is more beneficial, wherein the teacher asks direct questions and responds to a client's specific question attentively.

Teaching a mindfulness practice to those who have never experienced it before requires a little explanation, so that clients feel comfortable and secure, safe in the knowledge of what's to come and with an understanding of the teacher's role and how they will guide the practice.

I also explain the importance of inquiry and why it is a fundamental part of the practice and the client's learning. I describe the benefits derived from this process, without being outcome-focused or too specific about what I will be inquiring about. Informing clients that inquiry (exploring what happened through dialogue) helps the investigative process, brings clarity through an appreciation of the process.

The experience and knowledge of clients coming on mindfulness courses has changed dramatically over the last five years. I used to spend quite some time explaining what mindfulness is and what I mean by practice. The majority of people, most of whom self-select to attend, now have a good appreciation of these aspects, perhaps having read a book or two or listened to podcasts or apps. However, inquiry is still something of a mystery, mainly because this cannot usually be experienced by reading a book or starting to try to do it on your own. The profound benefit of being taught face to face, preferably either one-to-one or in smallish groups, is that the teacher can guide inquiry with every individual, working with their unique experiences. The acknowledgement, therefore, that inquiry may be an entirely new skill to learn and might take some time and application to acquire, supports engagement with the process. For some, trying to connect with and then find words to describe experiences is as challenging as learning a foreign language.

The process builds resources and, as we speak more slowly than we think, it puts everything into slow motion, giving time and space to investigate and process information that otherwise might have passed by so fleetingly, it would have gone unnoticed. It also provides the opportunity to watch how the experience unfolded and what the outcome was, creating the opportunity for learning and the development of insights and wisdom.

To put practice and inquiry into context, if the practice is relatively short, I would suggest spending about a third of the time before the practice explaining the rationale for doing it, what the practice entails and how long it will take. Approximately a third of the time is then taken in guiding the practice and another third in leading an inquiry afterwards.

For example, if I'm leading an abdominal breathing practice for ten minutes, I might take time at the outset to explain why this practice is helpful, saying how to pay attention to the belly, the chosen object, whether moving or still, that we're not trying to change anything, and also giving instructions as to what to do with a wandering mind. I might also describe a little of the anatomy and physiology and run through the importance of posture and loose clothing, as well as the ways in which breathing can be affected over time.

Throughout the practice, these instructions would be reaffirmed, with clear guidance on maintaining natural breathing, and an invitation towards the end to explore whether the clients' experiences have changed from when they first started the practice, without them having tried to elicit change. It can be quite a revelation to recognise that change has sometimes occurred without effort or will.

Followed by inquiry, therefore, guiding a relatively short practice may well take up to half an hour for someone who is new to mindfulness. As time goes by and appreciation of what mindfulness is, how to practice and the core features become more embedded, there is significantly less need to spend time on explanation prior to practice. The time given to inquiry, though, may well increase as more connections are being made, curiosity is piqued and understanding is deepened.

As practices lengthen and the client needs less practice instruction, this formula adjusts to about 50/50. Fifty per cent of the time is given to practice and the rest to inquiry. The learning from each of these elements can be profound and necessitates this time to explore and investigate experiences fully.

When working with a group, this timescale can be extended as the participants may all wish to share their experiences and this will inevitably spark further conversations about how mindfulness can become more deeply embedded in their lives.

Rather like race horse trainers who study past camera footage of how their horse moved, the position it took, the jockey's expertise and the going of the ground, the teacher can guide clients via the repetition of practices and exploration of the effects over time, thereby consolidating and expanding learning.

Intimately public and publicly intimate

Working one-to-one with a client ensures that inquiry dialogue flows from the teacher to the client and back again unimpeded.

Sometimes inquiry (either one-to-one or within a group setting) can be a very intimate process for both the client and the teacher. Of course, this is all set against the backdrop, within a group, of being conducted in a public domain. That is why it is essential that all clients have agreed their own group contracts at the beginning of the course, relating to confidentiality and what to do if someone becomes distressed.

The teacher needs to be able to maintain a balance, through awareness, of the individual client with whom they're dialoguing, as well as the others in the room who are all witnessing, by default, a very intimate exchange between two people.

Although the teacher may be inquiring with just one client, the others are not sitting there simply staring into space; they are also processing what they are witnessing and relating it to their own experiences. This can be a very moving and valuable experience for the engaged onlookers.

As familiarity with the inquiry process grows, the whole group may well be contributing to the process initiated by one client, and all aspects of the process are held, guided and overseen gently but firmly by the teacher.

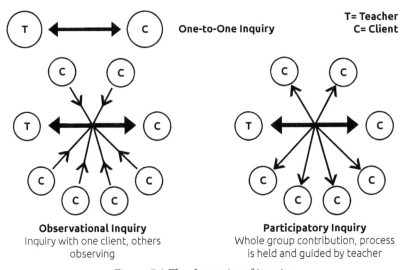

One-to-One Inquiry

T= Teacher
C= Client

Observational Inquiry
Inquiry with one client, others observing

Participatory Inquiry
Whole group contribution, process is held and guided by teacher

Figure 5.1 The dynamics of inquiry.

The language of inquiry

In Chapter 4 we explored the importance of being aware of ingrained, habitual language from a personal and/or professional context. Consideration of the power of language is imperative as it has such a major impact on the inquiry process.

Even the emphasis can affect the meaning. Consider the following, where the emphasis is placed on different words within the same sentence:

Mindfulness enriches your life.
Mindfulness *enriches* your life.
Mindfulness enriches *your* life.
Mindfulness enriches your *life*.

Connecting with emotions through language

Many people have a very limited amount of words to describe how they feel, particularly when describing emotions. Everything often just seems an emotional jumble, without any clarity, which can be overwhelming. The teacher can help clients to identify these feelings, through exploring more deeply what they are experiencing and then giving a choice of words that may relate to these feelings. For example, it's very common for a client to say after a practice that they feel really "nice". If the teacher inquires further into what "nice" means for them and they are unable to express it more eloquently, often a new teacher may leave it at that. Supporting clients to develop awareness of the more subtle and nuanced aspects of sensations and emotions, through the development of descriptive language, helps clients to become more in touch with their experiences, on a moment-by-moment basis.

Learning, through dialogue, to identify the emotions brings their understanding into the cognitive realm, thereby providing the opportunity to change the way they think and behave, which will impact on their ability to regulate their emotions more effectively.

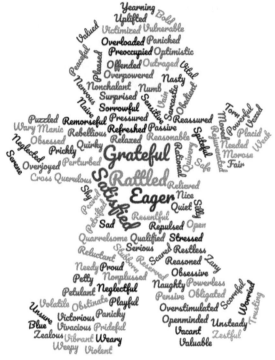

Figure 5.2 Connecting with emotions through language.

It may even be that the teacher has a list of the words in Figure 5.2 and asks the client to choose any that reflect their experiences, without imposing their own interpretations onto the client's emotional responses.

The power of language

When working with clients in other contexts, teachers might use some of the following words to give instructions or support clients, perhaps to elicit change:

analysing	clasping
balancing	contracting
building	controlling
changing	developing
considering	digging deep

distracting	reaching
explaining	reflecting
extending	relaxing
flexing	releasing
imagining	remembering
increasing	shortening
lengthening	stretching
moving	taking
pressing	thinking
producing	twisting
projecting	visualising

Mindfulness language

It can take some time to feel comfortable using mindful language and, when a new teacher feels a little anxious, these words can become elusive. The core features, intentions and attitudes of mindfulness can be taught and reinforced through the choice of words used, both when guiding practices and conducting inquiry. For example:

accepting	contacting
acknowledging	deepening
attention	embodying
attentive	examining
awareness	experiencing
being with	exploring
body sensations	feeling
choosing to rest	intuitively
compassionate	kindly
connecting	lean into

letting be	relating to
letting go	responding
light touch	resting
non-judgement	returning
not striving	sensing
observing	shining a light
patience	supporting
perspective	trusting
playfully	turn towards
present moment	understanding

Consider the phrase "letting go". Teachers often use this at the beginning of guiding a practice and it can be interpreted in a number of ways. The teacher may mean letting go of attention on external distractions, but the client might interpret it as "relaxing". The client's interpretation may have the effect of encouraging a letting go of attention, losing alertness and awareness – the antithesis of practice. Therefore the teacher must stay vigilant to their words, phrases, tone, inflections and other aspects of language that may be misinterpreted by the client to mean something else entirely.

Compassionate language

Similarly, compassionate language has its own subtleties and nuances and the teacher needs to consider when these words could be introduced to enhance the client's learning and experiences. For example:

caring	gently
courageously	giving
easing	gratitude
enabling	honouring
friendliness	kindness

listening to	self-compassion
nurturing	self-soothing
open-hearted	sensitively
receiving	softness
respecting	taking time
resting	tenderly
savouring	vulnerability

When the client is ready, the teacher starts introducing the concept of kindness and softness in relation to mindfulness practice and inquiry, so that it becomes familiar. I liken this to dropping in pearls of kindness, the teacher using language that enables the integration of their mindfulness practice experience with the attitude of kindness. Mindfulness is often taught like a plain, dry rice cracker, but kindness adds flavour, texture, substance and a heartiness to the experience.

Thus, adapting the language used according to the individual or group is essential, ensuring that they understand and appreciate the instructions, questions and guidance, whatever their age, background, skills and previous knowledge. Judging the level at which to teach is a skill that comes with practice.

Creating space with language

Being overwhelmed by thoughts and emotions can lead to the sense of being out of control or completely submerged within experiences. During inquiry, a teacher can create space with a simple change in language that completely changes perspective.

For example, after a breathing practice, the teacher may inquire, "What did you notice about your breath?" This engenders a personal association with the experience of the breath, with a sense of ownership implied. Alternatively, the teacher may ask, "What did you notice about the breath?" The word "the" replaces "your", thereby creating a sense of space and lessening personal identification. This is so very helpful in guiding clients to create perspective and to non-identify with physical sensations, emotions and thoughts. One word can create such a shift.

Another example is to explore the different experiences arising when relating to the body. If a client is experiencing pain, instead of asking, "What happened to your pain during the practice?", which implies ownership and attachment, replace "your" with "the". Pain then becomes a separate entity rather than all-consuming or part of the client's identity. It becomes another "thing" that feels more manageable and not inherently part of their being, thereby giving them the opportunity to approach and relate to it in an entirely different and healthier manner.

Finding their own truth through language

A client may ask a question about their experience during the practice and a teacher may swiftly and readily provide an answer. Another choice, if it feels pertinent, is to pause and let the question hang in the air for a while. Once it's landed and percolated, the client may say something along the lines of, "Ah, I think I might know the answer without you telling me". This is such a wonderful example of the effectiveness of talking about their experiences. Once the client has asked a question about their experience, it creates the opportunity to be "seen" and considered, without any verbal input from the teacher, though they have played a major part in the process. It's an extraordinary process and one not to be underestimated or rushed.

Getting started with inquiry

After a practice, clients are often more sensitive and open, resulting in a feeling of vulnerability as defences are softened around thoughts and feelings. Therefore the teacher needs to be kind, humble and have a genuine curiosity throughout the process of inquiry.

There is no "prescriptive" way of initiating inquiry; however, some considerations around how to start this process can be addressed, and there are some tricks of the trade.

Intentionality was discussed in Chapter 1, and this creates an excellent environment for starting the ball rolling, opening with relevant questions around clients' experiences, specifically in relation to these practices.

The teacher starts by asking open questions, rather than closed questions that require a "yes", "no" or one-word answer. This gives the opportunity for clients to explore rather than shut down their experiences. Saying something in the beginning such as, "I'd be really interested to hear your experiences of that practice", rather than, "Did you enjoy that experience?", will trigger the client's curiosity too.

If silence ensues, then asking them to turn to their neighbour to chat about a specific aspect (for example, whether they noticed any differences between how they felt in their body at the beginning, compared with the end of the body scan) can initiate dialogue. After inviting them to talk for three to five minutes, the teacher may then ask them to tell the group about their most noticeable experience. Alternatively, asking them to choose three words to explain how they felt is a quicker way for the teacher to get a sense of what happened for each person during the practice.

If the intention of the session is, for example, investigating patterns of thought, the teacher may have written common ones on pieces of paper and dotted them on the floor around the room. These may include the clients thinking about what they did earlier (remembering), wondering if they've got this right (judging), catastrophising about the future, and daydreaming or thinking about something like work or food. The teacher could then invite people to go to the thought pattern that was most prevalent during the three-minute practice that has just been led. Getting clients to move around like this often has the effect of starting a conversation.

Another technique is for the teacher to comment on what they observed, either in themselves or others. Maybe say something like, "I noticed tension in my throat. Did anyone else notice they were holding tension anywhere and, if so, what was that like?"

As the client or group starts to become familiar with the process, inquiry flows after each practice more readily, vocabulary begins to develop and understanding expands.

If working within a group context, inquiry with an individual could be quite fleeting; perhaps they simply need an acknowledgement of the experiences to reassure them that they are on the right track. Others need longer, with more time to investigate and pauses to deepen into the next awareness that is bubbling up, as they deal with more complex thoughts, feelings or emotions that arise. On average, an inquiry would take up to five minutes with one individual, though occasionally it may be longer.

Working one-to-one is very different. Inquiry might last a lot longer, usually moving from one aspect to another, as dictated by the client, enabling them to explore and investigate their experiences more fully and personally.

Disengaging from inquiry

When a teacher needs to move on, for whatever reason (perhaps to listen to another client's experience, teach another practice, deliver a teaching or reading, or because they are reaching the end of the session), a number of techniques can be employed to round things up.

I always acknowledge what has been said by either saying, "Thank you", or something similar, such as, "That sounds really helpful for you and perhaps it's something to reflect upon over the forthcoming week," or, "That's useful and I'd like to give it more time to discuss, so we'll come back to that in more detail on another session. Do you mind if we collectively hold that thought for now?" Other phrases I might use are as follows:

- That flows beautifully into what we're looking at next.

- That must have taken some courage to investigate and perhaps it's a good place to leave it for now.

- Why don't we just pause here and do a practice?

- Perhaps try using mindfulness the next time you notice that and tell us how you got on.

- I think someone else may have something to contribute too.

- That has been such a useful contribution but it's time to move on!

Using the body can be extremely helpful. Just turning away from one person towards the next one who wants to speak, dropping eye contact or closing down the posture can bring the process to an end.

Choosing which path to travel

Throughout the process of inquiry, a client, whether consciously or subconsciously, will choose which experience to feed back, and the teacher must discern which path of inquiry to travel down. Often, during feedback, a client might talk about a whole range of experiences, such as how things kept changing, or that they felt annoyed with themselves because they couldn't stay focused and they kept thinking about what they had to do tomorrow, which was causing them anxiety. A teacher needs to learn to regulate themselves as to which aspect to respond to: the nature of impermanence, acceptance, self-compassion, what to do with a wandering mind or the power of remaining present, in this example.

Having listened carefully to what and how the client is feeding back, the teacher chooses which path to take based on a whole range of factors, including:

• What the teacher senses in their own body when the client is feeding back. It can sometimes feel like a moment of clear attention, of connection, a sense of "That's it!"

• The context in which inquiry is being guided.

• What the teacher thinks would be the most helpful learning for the client.

• How aware the client is and whether they are ready for a particular learning at this stage.

• What would be of most benefit for the rest of the group?

• Whether the teacher feels confident and competent to explore a specific pathway.

• The time factor. It may be that the session is about to finish and there isn't sufficient time to explore the experience in depth.

• The client's own resources.

• The most relevant point in relation to the session or intention of the practice, teaching or course.

• Whether the choice relates to the needs of the teacher, who wants to hear more as it's juicy or relevant to them in some way. That choice might be in conflict with what the client needs to focus upon.

For example, following a mindful movement practice, a client may comment, "I noticed that I was able to pay attention to how I was feeling in this practice, more than any other we have done before, but that meant that my pain increased at the beginning." Some inquiry options for me would be:

- "What was it like for you to pay attention more fully during this practice?" This would help the client deepen their understanding of what it feels like to pay attention, moment-by-moment, and how beneficial this can be when suffering with pain.

- "What exactly did you notice happen when your pain increased and what did you do with that?" The client may have talked about how this increased their anxiety, but they trusted the process and their body, so continued with the practice.

- "You say that your pain increased at the beginning [reflection]. How did this change for you during the practice?" An exploration of the core feature related to impermanence may be helpful, or an investigation of what resources the client has that changed their experience by the end, encouraging them perhaps to pay attention more often when pain arises, rather than trying to distract themselves from it or put a lid on it.

There really is no right or wrong path. What feedback presents is often a series of options arising from one very short comment from a client, and the teacher chooses to guide the inquiry in the most beneficial direction for them at that moment.

There are occasions when teaching and inquiring may be inappropriate for a client and there are a number of aspects to consider regarding the efficacy and viability of guiding a client through this process.

If, for example, one is teaching a short grounding practice to a large group of people, such as in a workplace setting, there is no real need to be overly concerned about assessing their suitability for teaching. This is because a short, one-off practice will probably have the effect of stimulating the parasympathetic nervous system, helping them to feel calmer and more present. The effects will be superficial, short-lived and, I'm sure, very much appreciated. The inquiry will be around the physiological effects, what has happened regarding thoughts and perhaps how this practice could be utilised as a stress-management tool periodically throughout the day. Therefore, the teaching and inquiry would be light, with no need to assess these participants. This is also largely the case for the myriad of widely available online practices that are accessed via apps.

However, if longer practices are to be taught, more particularly if they are being practised regularly, it is essential to take a different stance. Longer practices go deeper, peeling back the layers of defences and tapping into the subconscious mind. It is there that habits, patterns, difficulties and perhaps traumas from the past reside, necessitating a more skilled approach.

The assessment process

If the teacher is delivering a course, or taking the client through a process of teaching, rather than a one-off introduction, it is essential to assess each client, to a greater or lesser extent, prior to teaching. It may well be that during this assessment process concerns are raised and action needs to be taken. This may also impact on how the teacher leads the inquiry, giving more of an indication of the difficulties arising, so that inquiry can be beneficially directed towards ways of dealing with these difficulties.

Toby was sent a written assessment with a view to attending a course that I was delivering in his workplace. It all came back as fairly benign: there were no real difficulties, he was not overly stressed and had plenty of support at home to practice. There was a question at the bottom of the page around why he wanted to attend the course, which he left blank.

It is my policy never to rely solely on a written assessment when assessing suitability to attend a substantial course. I always contact clients personally in order to have a conversation, start building a relationship and give them the opportunity to ask questions.

I am so used to assessing clients that Toby's lack of response precipitated in me a sense of curiosity as to why he left this last question blank. At first he said it was an error, but as I persisted in asking him about it, he revealed that there was indeed something he needed to talk to me about. He said that he had recently been diagnosed with Parkinson's disease but he didn't want his peers to know. He and his wife were going through a really difficult time coming to terms with the diagnosis and they were seeing a counsellor as a consequence.

Although his HR managers knew and were supportive, Toby had not told any of his colleagues as he was not ready to do so yet. With this knowledge and by exploring his incapacity to concentrate and inability to sit for prolonged periods, I was able to offer Toby more support. He would send me an email if he'd had a bad week and I didn't place him in a position where he had to share an explanation with his colleagues around how his week had been. I observed that some weeks he was more tired than others and this was reflected in his practice frequency and ability to stay focused during the session.

Had I not assessed Toby at the beginning, I'm sure we both would have had a very different experience of each other as he progressed through the course. I was able to give him discreet support when it came to discussions within the group, modify the mindful movement practice, offer postural advice, and limit exploratory and potentially revealing conversation with him, without the others becoming alert to the situation. I involved him in the inquiry process but maintained a compassionate awareness regarding how much to ask and when to draw back. Consequently, Toby learnt how to deal with this difficult diagnosis and reported that it helped with the suffering he was experiencing.

Assessment questions

The assessment questions really are the beginning of the inquiry process; that is, getting to know the individual or group and gaining an insight into how they relate to their own experiences. How they respond will impact on how the teacher leads an inquiry with them as the teaching progresses.

The questions are related to a range of factors including the following:

- The level of teaching required.
- Delivery mode – is it a one-off introduction or a substantial course?
- How best to engage the client(s).
- The setting.
- Is the teacher working one-to-one or with a group?
- The intention of the teaching – its aims and objectives.

- Remits (for example, from HR in an organisation, perhaps to address transition).

- Specialist client groups.

- Potential modifications and creative thinking regarding delivery.

- The frequency and longevity of practices.

- Is there an expectation that clients will practice between teaching sessions?

- Is there support away from the teaching sessions to practice?

- The age of the client(s).

- Is there any previous experience of mindfulness?

- Is the teaching purely mindfulness or is it combined with other teaching content?

- The size of the group.

- Mode of teaching, including face-to-face, blended, online.

- Ability to access support, such as whether the client(s) can download practices.

In the Appendix I have provided a couple of examples of assessments. One is the initial assessment I send to participants within an organisation, which I follow up with a more detailed face-to-face or telephone assessment. The other, I complete working one-to-one with clients with complex histories. They are there as examples, but I devise different assessments for different scenarios.

If possible, I would always strongly advocate a chat, usually no more than ten minutes per group participant, either on the phone or in person, unless their history is complex and more time is required to ensure safety and competence. When seeing a client one-to-one, the assessment often takes longer than ten minutes.

If this is not possible, then a group orientation session may be an option. This gives clients the opportunity to complete a health questionnaire or assessment tool, to be repeated at the end of the course to monitor outcomes. These tools or scales may measure levels of stress, mindfulness and self-compassion, anxiety and depression, propensity to ruminate, sleep patterns, general health and wellbeing, or any other aspects the teacher wishes to monitor.

COMPASSIONATE MINDFUL INQUIRY IN THERAPEUTIC PRACTICE

Once these assessment questions have been collated and analysed, they inform the teacher more clearly how best to construct the programme to reflect individual needs and those of the group as a whole.

During the assessment process, the teacher may ask some or all of the following questions:

- General questions relating to contact details including name, address, phone number, email address.

- GP and contact details, if appropriate.

- Where they heard about the mindfulness course (for example, referral, HR, website).

- Presenting physical, psychological and/or emotional difficulties – in particular, levels of stress, anxiety, pain or depression.

- Recent difficult life events such as bereavement, divorce, redundancy or other significant change.

- Medication and its effects.

- Recreational drug use and alcohol consumption.

- Past medical/psychological history.

- Suicidality, psychosis, PTSD, acute depression, severe social anxiety.

- Family, work, group support.

- Current treatment/therapy (for example, cognitive behavioural therapy).

- Perception of amount of spare time to do the home practice, if given.

- Client's expectations.

- Sleep – insomnia, chronic fatigue syndrome, sleep hygiene.

- Language and communication skills – does the client need an interpreter, sign language or loop system for hearing aid?

- Educational/intellectual understanding will determine how the information is pitched.

- Past experience in meditation, yoga, mindfulness.

- Any other support they may require to ensure they get the most from the teaching.

- Requirements for mats, blocks, cushions, blankets, chairs.

During the assessment or orientation session, the teacher may explain the following:

- What the course entails – number of sessions, timings, rules around absenteeism, certificates, course content and contact details.

- The importance of home practice – explore how they would fit this into their daily life.

- The challenges of the course, turning inwards, increasing awareness, being with suffering.

- Exploring whether they are currently experiencing significant changes or life events.

- The support system available to them outside of the course (from the teacher, colleagues, resources or others), if necessary.

- The experiential aspects, emphasising the need for personal reflection and openness.

- How many are in the group, the venue, details regarding parking, clothing, payment, what to bring (include information on any retreat element at this stage, if this is being offered).

- Issues regarding confidentiality, familiarity with other members of the group and the impact this may have.

- Explain that if the teacher has significant concerns, they may contact the GP or other professional, with the client's consent.

- If there are going to be other teachers offering co-teaching, videoing classes, observing, teacher supervision or anyone else in the room.

- That they might be asked to do some pair work and additional exercises in class, which may be shared.

Most people do not attend a mindfulness course when everything in their life is going well, so the majority of clients will be experiencing some difficulties, to a greater or lesser extent. Therefore, the teacher needs to know when to delve a little deeper to determine whether it's safe for the client to attend or whether it's more appropriate to signpost them to another professional.

Feeling uneasy

I am often asked by my supervisees what to do if the teacher feels uneasy or doesn't think that an individual should attend. There's no straightforward answer to this, but I inquire into the following with them:

- Is this participant triggering something in you – perhaps from your own past experiences – that leads you to feel uneasy?

- Is there anything else you can ask to gain more insight into this situation?

- Is there anyone else you can talk to about them confidentially, such as HR?

- What exactly is the nature of the difficulty?

- With additional support, such as supervision, will you feel supported enough to teach them?

- What is your intuition telling you?

- Is there anything else you can do to create more of a sense of safety for you or the client?

- How do you think it would be for the client to talk with them about waiting a while to start this process?

Ultimately my advice to a teacher is to trust their gut instincts, but the teacher can't just say that they're not going to teach them. I would say something like:

It's been really useful talking to you about your wish to learn mindfulness. My sense is that this is not quite the right time for you, so I would recommend you chat to your GP/HR about your difficulty and come back to me in the future. How does that sound?

The important aspect here is that teaching mindfulness and leading inquiry is part of an educational process – getting to know the self more fully – and should not be approached by either the teacher or client as a therapy.

Potential red flags

Mindfulness teaching and inquiry are sometimes not suitable for an individual. There are few real hard-and-fast rules and the decision ultimately lies within the teacher's own skill set and the setting in which they're working. I have certainly taught mindfulness and led successful inquiries with people for whom, on paper, it would be contraindicated. I made this informed choice due to my experience and clinical background, and closely monitored the effects throughout the process.

The assessment process is imperative to flag up any difficulties that may preclude mindfulness teaching and inquiry as an intervention, and whether teaching may potentially cause more problems and/or an exacerbation of the client's symptoms and levels of distress. Aligned with this is asking clients whether they have ever practised mindfulness before and determining the effects of these experiences. The responses to this question may require further investigation as to how they were taught, what the practices were and their duration.

Below are some guidelines and rationales to help a teacher make that choice. Even though a teacher may not be leading an in-depth inquiry afterwards, the act of practising mindfulness meditations culminates in self-inquiry, going deeper. This self-inquiry can precipitate change, which may be destabilising. Therefore, the teacher needs to consider whether the participant is well-enough resourced and has enough stability and support to deal with whatever arises appropriately and safely.

A teacher may have many hats that they wear and feel competent within their professional field, but it is necessary when teaching mindfulness to stay within the boundaries of a mindfulness teacher, which may be a whole new role for them. The teacher's competency must therefore be considered, especially with regard to leading inquiry.

When teaching specialist clients or groups, it is essential that the teacher is well-informed about the participants' area of expertise, in order to be aware of the challenges and know how to adjust teaching and modify inquiry to suit their clients' needs appropriately. Teachers must also have the right support themselves, have regular supervision, consider their own safety and that of others, and ensure that they are fully insured to deliver the practices and lead inquiry.

Acute and chronic illnesses

Much of the original research conducted on the benefits of mindfulness is with clients suffering with chronic conditions. Indeed, Jon Kabat-Zinn (2013) developed the MBSR programme for people with long-term health problems.

It may be that if a client has an acute illness or exacerbation of a chronic illness, this is not an appropriate time to partake in learning mindfulness. For example, during a flare-up of a physical condition or an acute episode of a mental health problem, other forms of intervention may be more appropriate.

Only those professionals working within mental health should teach mindfulness to clients who are suffering with clinical levels of anxiety, depression or other mental health problems. Clients need to be assessed thoroughly to determine whether mindfulness is appropriate at this time. Teaching should be delivered by highly trained mental health professionals who are supported within the healthcare setting and system.

Suicidal ideation

Clients presenting with suicidal ideation are extremely vulnerable. It is, therefore, of paramount importance that clients receive the appropriate support from highly skilled professionals and must be signposted immediately.

Life crises

As a very general rule, those clients who have recently experienced bereavement, a difficult health diagnosis or trauma may be advised not to practice mindfulness or to attend a course at this time. It may be more helpful to offer them the teaching once the emotionally charged event has stabilised and the client is in a better place to learn new coping strategies and practices. Teaching should then be regulated and adjusted to suit the client's needs.

Substance misuse

This includes both drug and alcohol misuse. Clients will be unlikely to take part in any mindfulness teaching if under the influence of either substance as their ability to stay present and develop awareness will be compromised. However, a Mindfulness-Based Relapse Prevention course (Bowen, Chawla & Martlatt 2010) has been developed for this client group and is delivered by skilful, knowledgeable teachers with a background of working in this field.

Psychosis and severe mental health problems

Mindfulness is generally contraindicated for clients suffering with psychosis and severe, acute mental health problems. This is because their diagnosis indicates that they are out of touch with reality, and mindfulness is based on recognising the reality of the situation to gain perspective. However, if clients are stabilised on medication and have the full support of their mental health teams, mindfulness, particularly in the form of mindful movement in conjunction with a compassionate attitude, may be helpful.

Early trauma, past abuse, post-traumatic stress disorder and dissociative disorders

Mindfulness can either help or hinder clients with these difficulties, depending on the events themselves, their level of support and the stage of recovery. I believe that teaching by people who are not sufficiently trained, in addition to an inappropriate teaching context, such as a retreat setting, is at the root of much of the negative press around the teaching of mindfulness. Again, this aptly demonstrates the need for understanding, skill and caution in assessing the client and delivering mindfulness to these vulnerable individuals. I applaud conversations regarding the appropriateness and efficaciousness of teaching and inquiring as it demonstrates the importance of teaching by skilled, trained teachers who have professional experience of these clients.

It is true that some clients sign up to a course, possibly without having told the teacher of their past, or even having a conscious memory of what they have experienced. This is one reason I make it very clear that this is an education programme and not therapy, though it clearly is a therapeutic approach to healing processes.

The teacher must be constantly vigilant for changes in clients as teaching progresses. If they are seeing clients over weeks and months, life events that are completely unrelated to the course may destabilise the clients.

On occasion, a client may describe a sensation of "leaving the body" during practice. This can be a mental or spiritual experience, but it may also be a dissociative defence mechanism, whereby the memories of trauma are too painful or dangerous to face. Embodiment practices may be contraindicated, so teaching practices that invite paying attention to objects some distance from the body or practising mindful movement or mindful walking can help to ground and stabilise the client.

Post-traumatic stress disorder (PTSD) may well be restimulated by mindfulness because of the space created, tapping into the sub-conscious mind and being given the opportunity to reconnect with the deeply emotional event. The client may not have the necessary resources for this at the time, so an alternative, supportive intervention may be more appropriate.

If the trauma was a sexual assault, clients will need expert support, and mindfulness teaching should only be delivered by experienced professionals working in this field.

Unwittingly, the teacher may trigger extreme emotional responses. It is, therefore, essential to be constantly vigilant, teaching and inquiring in small doses – titrating the dose, as Steve Hickman[1] explains on the Mindful Self-Compassion Teacher Training programme. The teacher must be constantly monitoring the effects of teaching over time.

If a client does express that they are experiencing trauma in response to a practice, there are a number of questions I might ask to determine whether it's appropriate for them to continue. I would be interested to know what aspect of the practice triggered their

---

1   Personal communication (2019) with Steve Hickman (Executive Director of the Centre for Mindful Self-Compassion).

emotional response. If, for example, the trauma was specifically related to the neck and during a body scan practice attention here stimulated an emotional reaction, the teacher might simply advise the client to avoid bringing attention to this area, or to proceed with a different practice. If the client was able to physically remain in the room, highlighting the resources that enabled them to do this builds confidence and courage. Introducing other mindful devices such as counting the breaths has the effect, for some, of lessening the emotional reaction by giving the client something else as their primary object. Finally, asking what happens if they are able to bring kindness and self-soothing to the experiences can facilitate a "holding" of the experience rather than a resistance and aversion to it.

These recommendations are given to those teachers who are equipped to support the client fully and should not be undertaken by anyone new to teaching or without the expertise and experience to guide inquiry safely.

Breathing difficulties

Participants suffering with breathing problems, such as asthma, may find that using their breath as an anchor is unhelpful. It may be that guiding them to use another part of their body as their safe place would be beneficial, particularly lower in the body, to ground them. It can also be useful to instruct them to think of the air just beyond their nose or just at the tip of their nostrils so that they are still working with the breath, but it is focused outwardly and not internally. Of course, if the client is full of cold then advising them to do another practice such as the body scan, or breathe through their mouth, may be more beneficial.

Dealing with challenges

Clients in a group setting usually speak up, or interject in some way, for one of three reasons: they need to be heard, for whatever reason; there was a problem or conflict within the practice; the problem is still there and they need support and advice around unpacking this and developing resources to build into their "what next".

The latter two reasons are easier to address through skilful teaching and inquiry. Often the first one manifests in a huge variety of ways and takes real skill and experience to manage – for the sake of the teacher, the client and the other group participants, equally. Some of these presentations are explored below.

Being taught in this experiential way is an alien situation for most people, so there is often initially some stress and anxiety around the whole process. It is quite likely that clients will revert to their own default mode as they are subconsciously reminded of their school days or childhood (for example, they may become talkative or quiet, make little eye contact, raise their hand to ask a question, giggle, form a clique or want to rebel). As these feelings of unease subside, clients start to investigate and explore this uncharted territory with more confidence.

My aim here is not to pigeon-hole people – we're all beautifully unique – but to address specific presentations and, hopefully, offer some guidance about certain techniques to deal with these challenges as they arise when leading inquiry.

I would say that I generally try to address the situation in class but on occasion I have asked people to stay behind or contacted them between sessions to talk to them about the effect their conduct is having on the group dynamics and teaching process. In these situations I invite them to become more aware of their habits around communication and this often leads to considerable insights.

Talkative

The teacher may well have led a practice and asked the group to share their experiences of that practice. Often it's the same person – the talkative one – who always pipes up first. There are pros and cons to them as they often get the ball rolling and lead others to find their voice, but they can also set the tone of the inquiry, guiding the discussion in a domineering way. The teacher must notice, too, what arises in themselves when someone else does much of the talking.

Sometimes being talkative is a defence mechanism and the person settles down after a couple of sessions when they feel less anxious. Others may just like the attention or have something significant going on in their lives that they'd like to explore there and then. However, some people really do suffer from verbal diarrhoea and this needs to be addressed.

Whatever the reason, it is perfectly alright for the teacher to interject, perhaps acknowledging what's being observed by saying something like, "It seems that you have a lot to say about this. Is it OK if I just ask you one thing about your experience?" The teacher can perhaps make an observation such as, "As you are talking, I can see your body becoming agitated. Could you please show me with your hand where you feel it the most?" This has the effect of bringing them out of thinking, sometimes a state of being overwhelmed, to the physical sensations, thereby changing the dynamics and helping to ground them.

Synonymous with this presentation is the storyteller. Whilst stories can be very entertaining and enrich the course, some people are like professionals and need to be curtailed from time to time. Expanding upon James's comments in Chapter 1, about the "root" being the important thing in what a client is saying, rather than their actual words, the teacher can bring the conversation back by asking questions such as, "In which part of the practice did you notice your thoughts going into the story?", "What happened to take you from being in the practice to thinking about the story", or "What would it be like for you, when you start going into the story, to bring your awareness back to the here and now?" The analogy extends further in that the propensity for storytelling can be likened to a rambling vine that has roots anchoring to the wall or ground for stability. The teacher is interested in these roots, the core features, habits, mind traps or whatever, rather than the actual content of the story itself.

When leading inquiry, I might say something like, "Thank you for sharing that. It would be really interesting to hear if anyone else felt the same, or indeed very differently", so that I turn their volume down, rather like a radio, and turn my attention elsewhere.

Following a practice, I might want another client to be given the opportunity to speak first. Therefore, although the teacher should never specifically ask a particular person what their experience was, I might say, "X often speaks first during inquiry and it would be great to hear from someone else first this time."

Sometimes there are two competitors in the room, vying for the limelight, and this can be challenging. One person may say something and the next ramps it up a bit and describes a "bigger and better" experience and so it goes on. The teacher really must intervene for the benefit of the whole group, maybe inviting time to pause before the next person speaks or, even better, going into another mini practice that explores emotions or communication processes.

Inviting clients to give just one to three words to describe their experiences can help to curtail those who have more to say, and something like "Let's just have one more comment before we move on" creates boundaries and prevents others from joining in. The teacher could suggest that clients consider whether what they're about to say is a conscious contribution. By this I mean that before speaking they reflect on whether their inquiry feedback is useful for themselves or anyone else in the group. It's also a good idea to reiterate that inquiry relates to the experience within the practice and the application of mindfulness in everyday life, as a way of preventing too much wandering off the point and bringing them back to the intention of mindfulness.

Very quiet or silent

Within a group there are often a few people who are quieter, more reserved. The teacher's role is to guide and support everyone equally, so it's important to notice if a client hasn't contributed much to the inquiry process.

We all process information in different ways; some people are more internally reflective than others. Just because a client isn't contributing doesn't mean they're not getting anything out of listening to other people during inquiry. However, what they are missing out on is the opportunity to explore their own experiences that arise from practice and perhaps to make links to habitual patterns that a teacher, as a skilled observer, may be able to identify more readily.

There is something very powerful about verbalising an experience – getting it out into the ether, so to speak, so that it can be acknowledged fully.

Of course, it may well be that the client is incredibly shy and the teacher should not put them in a position in which they feel extremely exposed by asking them a question directly. However, it's helpful to enable them to find their voice, if they so wish, and contribute to the conversations that arise within a group as part of inquiry. One way to support this is to ask clients to get into pairs to chat about their experiences. They then come back to the group and each person shares one or two things that have been discussed in relation to the practice or course content. When the quiet one speaks, ask more questions, perhaps broadening the question to other aspects of the course that have already been covered to get a sense of where they are. This is often enough to open the dialogue a little. The following week, you might then say something relating to what they had spoken about the week before and fold it into the next layer of learning.

Maggie had not spoken at all in the first half of the mindfulness course and hadn't made eye contact with anyone, so I quietly asked her at the end of session three if she had a couple of minutes to stay behind for a quick chat. I said that I had noticed that she was very quiet and asked if there was anything I could do to support her further on the course. She told me that she felt very anxious and that by the time she had plucked up the courage to say anything, someone else had started talking.

We explored what we could do together, and she asked if she could sit next to me in the circle so she didn't have to make direct eye contact with me but could feel my presence; in that way she felt more comforted. She said that if she had something to say she'd lean towards me a little and I could ask her if she had anything on her mind. Maggie also said she enjoyed the pauses as they gave her space to plan what she was going to say more clearly and she felt a lot less rushed. During the second half of the course she gained confidence and contributed much more to the process of inquiry. She no longer needed to gesture with her body before speaking, and inquiry started to arise quite naturally.

But what if no one speaks? How long does a teacher leave it before they break the silence? I have the capacity, as a teacher, to hold a silence for ages but I am acutely aware of others squirming and becoming embarrassed. It's very exposing, talking about thoughts and emotions in a circle of strangers without a desk or anything to hide behind.

In these circumstances I'd go back into pair work or ask very specific questions, perhaps relating to my own experiences arising from the practice, such as, "My hands started to feel really warm during that practice. Did anyone else notice that, or did you feel the opposite?" Temperature is something that most of us can relate to and it often starts a conversation flowing.

Sometimes the teacher needs to feed the response or resource to clients by asking, "Would it help if...?" or "Perhaps you could consider..." This gives them something to relate to so that they learn more of the languaging around their experiences and gain an understanding of the direction they can go in beyond practice to enhance their lives.

Analytical

There are those that question everything, more especially at the beginning of the process. They require empirical and anecdotal evidence, perhaps asking if the teacher has ever experienced anyone like them before. Always going into intense thinking and rationalising prior to engagement can sometimes be a defence mechanism.

Several years ago, I saw a veterinary surgeon, Piers Pepperell,[2] who did just this. He found himself in a dark place, over-analysing, caught up in ruminations and catastrophic thoughts, which had a debilitating effect on his mood. Coming from a scientific background, he wanted to know why and how mindfulness worked, what my plan for him was and what the outcomes would be, with timescales. I answered his questions for a while so that he would become more comfortable, engaged and trusting of me and the whole process. However, the watershed came when he let go of his analytical mind and fully engaged with the practice, allowing himself to feel into the experiences and inquire into how these were mirrored in his own life. He began to build a more positive relationship with his body and mind, which had the life-changing effect of opening his heart. What a joy it was to witness this transformation, turning his life around, radiating joy and happiness, with an infectious zest for life that had once seemed completely beyond reach.

Often clients start off with thinking about what is happening rather than directly experiencing it; sometimes they have a narrative going on whilst practising. During a breath meditation, for example, they might be saying to themselves, "Now I'm feeling the breath going in and then there's a gaseous exchange and then I breathe out."

By becoming aware that this is their experience for them during practice, the teacher can repeatedly ask from one session to the next, "What does that experience of analysing and constant thinking feel like in the body?" Over time, usually, the analytical mind becomes more accepted as a mechanism for processing information, perhaps being seen as a protection device, and slowly a balance between this,

---

2   Personal communication (2019) with Piers Pepperell (veterinarian).

the sensations of the body and the emotions is experienced. The learning that arises from acknowledging that a client has an analytical mind can be quite a revelation as it may be that they have never had the forum to look at this before with another.

Tearfulness

When another person cries our mirror neurons fire off and we want to help. Other group members often attempt to rescue or "fix" the situation, but their efforts can be inappropriate. At the beginning of the course, even during the assessment process, I talk about what might happen in response to practice and inquiry, explaining that none of us can predict what will arise emotionally during this course. I show everyone the box of tissues at the beginning and explain the benefits of getting in contact with our own suffering – it's our point of change and growth. A friend of mine, Singhashri Gazmuri,[3] coined the phrase "resistance is fertile", and this recognition of how we've been resisting or suppressing a painful emotion can lead to tearfulness. I ask the group to resist their own urge to comfort, suppress or placate their fellow-client, and instead to give the individual space for distress and unease to arise, be seen and processed so that insights can permeate via their felt sense.

I then check in with the person who was distressed later in the session or during the week, giving the opportunity to talk further, should they wish to.

Controller

Control creates suffering, so this is a topic that arises frequently during inquiry. It can also mean that there is someone in the group who is very controlling of others and, occasionally, the teacher.

Some clients have a need to take ownership of some of the processes. This is exhibited by behaviour such as arriving too early so they can help set up, during which time they might have a quiet word about something; arriving late and causing a scene; needing to leave early, giving the impression that they're too important to be

---

3   Personal communication (2017) with Singhashri Gazmuri (mindfulness teacher and trainer).

able to spare the whole time; or maybe attempting to hang around afterwards, wanting to talk about other clients in the group.

The teacher needs to be awake to these behaviours and nip them in the bud as they can lead to feelings of unease, even distrust, from the rest of the group.

Competitiveness

One supervisee, Leah Callebaut,[4] described her experience of a group she was leading. One half of the group were new to mindfulness and the other half considered themselves experts in this field and wanted everyone to know it, thereby having the effect of splitting the group into two halves. The "experts" often stepped in, giving advice about meditation to the "newbies" and occasionally taking on the role of teacher. There was so much to inquire about with this scenario but, ultimately, the situation created difficulties. Those who were new to mindfulness felt their feelings and needs were being overlooked by the more vocal, eloquent and experienced half.

Setting out clear boundaries from the outset was advised for next time, giving the teacher the option of reminding the group about these should things get too challenging. By supporting the supervisee in developing a more fiercely compassionate attitude, balance and equilibrium were restored by the end of the course.

Lack of practice

We all have times, I'm sure, when practice eludes us. I particularly like the analogy of this being a marathon and not a sprint, and taking the long view is very helpful to me in supporting my own practice.

During the assessment process, the invitation to practice between teaching sessions is explored with the client, identifying times when they perceive they will be able to practice and any support they may need to ensure this is achieved.

However, and I feel like writing this in capitals, very often clients still say that they didn't realise there would be home practice and simply do not have time to do it. I play good cop/bad cop in this scenario. Firstly, I know how hard it is to find the time to develop a new habit and let go of old ones, but I am quite firm about the

---

4   Personal communication (2019) with Leah Callebaut (mindfulness teacher).

invitation to practice, citing brain changes to incentivise them. Often there is a honeymoon period at the beginning of teaching and clients are very engaged with their practice. As the brain starts to change, letting go of old habits, challenges may arise, manifesting as barriers to practice in a whole range of guises, and there is sometimes a wobble in the middle of a course, around weeks three, four and five.

Inquiry helps in identifying their barriers to practice, too, as there are often practical suggestions that a teacher can give that will support the client in finding the time and inclination to practice.

Exploring this propensity to not engage with practice can also be insightful for the client. It may reveal a lack of self-care, perhaps acknowledging that they like to fill every spare moment, or they have some other pattern from the past that prevents them beginning or continuing with their practice: procrastination.

There are often those that have taken up a fair bit of time explaining why they haven't practised and the teacher needs to ascertain when to say that it's up to them to decide whether they are able to make the most out of the teaching and their work together. Ultimately, the teacher is simply there to facilitate and guide the way and it's up to the client as to whether they take this on or not.

If it is clear that the client has tried hard but circumstances disallow their ability to practice for half an hour or so, I will suggest that they reduce the time to, say, ten minutes in the morning and ten minutes later in the day. Ensuring practice is manageable is crucially important in sustaining practice long-term. In this instance, I do believe that a little bit of something is better than a lot of nothing.

When working with a group, other clients' progress incentivises those who are slower to get off the mark with their practice. Changes can start to happen remarkably quickly, and others will wish to follow, stepping up the length or intentionality regarding practice.

Ensuring clients have the support they need to establish a reliable practice is crucial, and beyond this is the development of the skills and resources to be able to inquire into their experiences. This support may come in the form of guided practices, handouts, contact between sessions, shared forums to discuss difficulties and how to overcome challenges, signposting to other online resources, the instigation of a peer support model, meditation buddies or other creative mechanisms. Whatever is employed must be embedded with the intention of overcoming obstacles and enabling practice, learning and development to flourish in a non-judgemental and kindly way.

Increased pain

An increase in pain, be it physical, emotional or psychological, is very common at the beginning of practice and often much of inquiry is given towards explaining and investigating the role of mindfulness in managing these experiences. This can be quite challenging for the client as well as for others who may be listening and observing the dialogue, if it's a group setting.

When working one-to-one with a client's personal experiences in this domain, the inquiry process can be very beneficial from the outset, helping the client to describe their experiences, especially the subtle ones, and enabling them to appreciate the benefits of mindful attention when imbued with kindness. The teacher can progress at the right pace for the client and address any issues arising there and then.

That said, hearing within a group setting that others suffer too can have many positive effects on how a client relates to their pain. Certainly, their pain is physical, but it will also be having an emotional and psychological impact. Therefore it is extraordinarily powerful to listen to and experience the suffering of others who are working together as a group to find ways to manage suffering.

Awareness of suffering certainly softens the defence mechanisms. These defences have some benefits for clients and the teacher needs to recognise when these defences are serving to keep the client well. In the long term, these defence mechanisms tighten and contract around the suffering and serve only to increase suffering further. During inquiry, the identification of the presence of pain and exploring what the client does with it, how they relate to it and their relationship with it, in all its forms, is what leads to developing the capacity to lean into it with more kindness. By familiarising themselves with the experiences, reactions, behaviours and beliefs associated with their pain, a client can learn to manage it with more ease through kindly acceptance, while being guided and nurtured by the teacher.

Complaining clients

Clients may have a habit of complaining, perhaps about the programme, lack of progress, the process, practices, the teacher or others. Inquiry helps to identify these patterns and explores the possibility of change through being more mindful of their communication styles and exploring the impact this presentation has on themselves and others. Boundaries are extremely important from the start, and a compassionate teacher will help clients to identify and modify maladaptive behaviours, through skilful inquiry.

Learning modalities

When considering the needs of an individual or group, it may be helpful to consider how they would best engage with the practices so that the inquiry will be rich and fruitful. Although this viewpoint around learning modalities is somewhat outdated, and a combined approach is now accepted as more usual, it's true that we all learn in different ways at different times and the teacher must consider all learning styles so that there is something to support everyone's learning. It's also important for the teacher to recognise their own style as this is the one they will use and default to most in their teaching, although it won't be optimal for all.

I learn best via a combination of auditory and kinesthetic experiences, so I have to remind myself to draw an image or write on the board to support those who learn more through visual cues. Sometimes doing a mind map or using another device on the flipchart can be helpful when leading inquiry.

Achieving a balance with all three teaching styles when conducting inquiry is important (see Table 5.1).

Table 5.1 Teaching styles

Visual	Consider the use of graphs and drawings of the outline of the body for clients to identify where they felt sensations during practice. Practising a mountain meditation, or using pebbles or beautiful things as the objects of practice are all worth considering.
Kinesthetic	Asking questions about the sensations in the body and where emotions are felt after mindful movement, eating, touching and walking meditations can elicit deeper inquiry.
Auditory	Sound practices, listening to beautiful poetry, guided meditations and verbal presentations all support auditory learning. Inquiry is aided through conversation, in pairs or the whole group. The act of verbalising experiences helps clients to gain greater insight into what's going on for them in that moment.

Gaining clarity

Reflecting back to a client what was thought to have been understood from them about their feedback helps to validate what they say, relating to it from an open-hearted position. It can also be quite emotional for a client, hearing someone else say their own words back to them, reaffirming what they have experienced.

The teacher needs to be cautious about over-doing this technique as the client is the expert in their own experience and it can appear a little contrived and repetitive, blocking further investigation and inquiry.

Getting it wrong, whether it's reflecting back or another aspect of inquiry, happens quite a bit as a teacher. This may well be very uncomfortable for the teacher and they need to be alive to the internal reactions that arise when this happens. For example, saying something like, "I get a sense that you mean...", and the client responds with, "No, I didn't mean that at all". If this occurs, come back to it and say, "Thank you for letting me know that. Perhaps it would be helpful to explain it slightly differently, so I understand it better", rather than leaving them feeling unheard and misunderstood.

Ask permission regarding whether it's OK to go into an experience in more detail. This creates a sense of being in control as well as piquing their interest into what is really happening for them. I would say something like, "Would it be OK to explain that in a bit more detail to me, please, so that I can get a better understanding of how that is for you?"

If a client is clearly experiencing something tender, I would always ask permission to investigate further, acknowledging that this has the potential for an emotional charge but also has the potential to lead to change. I would say something like, "Is it OK if I ask you a little more about your experience, please, as it feels sensitive?" Of course, the client always has the opportunity to say "No" and this must be respected at all times.

Investigating delicate experiences takes courage, so I might make a comment about how that feels important for them or that it must take courage to look at things in that way, whatever it was. I would always then finish by saying, "Thank you". It is such a privilege to do this sensitive work – asking people to pull back the layers of their defences to expose the raw and vulnerable – and it feels absolutely appropriate to thank them for their trust in the teacher and the process.

Consideration of other significant factors will impact on how the teacher relates to the clients and them to each other.

Promoting a sense of connection

When a client enters a space to learn mindfulness and take part in inquiry, there may be a sense of feeling separate, arising from not knowing what to expect, meeting a new person or people for the first time, preconceived ideas about what this process might entail and an uncertainty about how much they are expected to partake and/or reveal about themselves. Connectivity and ease can be promoted in a number of ways.

Firstly, as mentioned in Chapter 4, arranging seating in a circle, in a group, or slightly off-set when working one-to-one, with the teacher as part of that circle, perhaps giving a little space on either side, means that clients feel more comfortable and there's no issue around sitting at the back or front in a classroom style. Conversation flows more readily as everyone is equal and can make eye contact with everyone else.

Inviting clients to move around, either within a session or from one session to the next, means that there's more connection via pair work and more opportunity for general chit-chat.

Consider ice-breakers, such as asking each person to share something that may be somewhat surprising or unexpected. This is a way of introducing humour and light-heartedness at the beginning and can allay fears and create warmth.

Sometimes even changing the whole room around, with the teacher sitting somewhere else, or leaving the room empty of chairs at the beginning of one session and starting with a walking practice, creates a sense of "we're all in this together". It can also highlight how quickly habits are formed and what occurs when they are disturbed.

In larger groups, where a circle may not be possible, it can be valuable to think creatively about the space – for example, the potential of getting people into smaller groups in their seating arrangements or having an assistant to take them to break-out rooms so that inquiry is more personal.

The nature of inquiry is just that – a personal experience – so consider whether it is necessary to give everyone the opportunity to contribute to the process. If there is a large number of people for one or two sessions, I would not deem this necessary. However, if the intention is to support people going deeper into their own experiences, then the largest group I would consider working with on my own is 16 people. As a starting suggestion, I would recommend 6–12 as ideal.

The use of props to enable comfort promotes a sense of community – for example, one person getting the equipment for the others, and everyone sitting there, perhaps with their feet on blocks – something that doesn't happen in other group scenarios. Using bolsters, zafus, mats, meditation stools, cushions and blankets all adds to the feeling of common humanity. By tapping into the client's own needs as well as those of others through the sharing of equipment, kindness pervades.

Seats should be relatively upright and supportive but not too rigid; the room should be clean and warm with reasonable lighting, quietish and uninterrupted; everyone needs to be able to see the flipchart or screen; refreshments, especially water, should be provided.

Each session may require different materials such as food and utensils for an eating meditation, pens and paper, envelopes, printed laminated cards, handouts, readings and exercise sheets, to promote learning and inquiry.

Teach what you know

It is essential that the teacher teaches what they know and feel comfortable with, as taking a client to this place of vulnerability is extremely therapeutic if handled with care but has the potential to cause difficulties if handled unskilfully, leaving the client feeling exposed and unresourced.

A teacher will be very aware of the terrain, but it's important to stay close to the sense that the clients are experts in their own experiences, so there truly is no right or wrong and no judgement. This is certainly an equal and mutual process of investigation and the teacher is the facilitator of this, especially at the beginning of the process.

Discernment

It's sometimes easy to get caught up in thinking that we should not be judging others whilst teaching. There is, however, a huge difference between being discerning and being judgemental.

Being discerning means staying alert to all that is going on within the room, remaining aligned with one's own teaching intentions and motivations, and making decisions and choices through skilful means.

For example, the teacher needs to discern whether they are going to focus in on one person's experience or open inquiry up to the whole group more fully, perhaps comparing and contrasting experiences. Maybe saying, "Thank you for sharing that. Did anyone else have similar or completely different experiences?" will stimulate discussions. I particularly like the concept of a torch beam. Sometimes it's helpful to keep the beam wide, general and soft, discussing experiences with the whole group; at other times it's appropriate to focus in sharply, shining a clear light on one person's experience and investigating that in depth, enabling them to see new possibilities emerging out of the darkness.

It is important to stay attuned to how clients are responding to this process and to discern whether they are open, in a place where they can experience good, emotional work, or closed and need to stay in a place of safety. Signs that clients are closed may be that they appear irritable, sleepy or disengaged. Let clients know that all of this is OK and that this teaching creates an environment in which they can take care of their own needs, whatever they may be in this moment.

A teacher can, therefore, synchronise a non-judgemental yet discerning attitude whilst teaching clients.

Phrases

Rather like poetry or readings, the use of phrases during inquiry can help to exemplify what is going on for a client. Some useful mindfulness and compassion phrases are as follows:

"What you resist persists"

This relates to a common way of dealing with difficulties, which in the short term can be a useful strategy but long-term is unsustainable. I liken it to a pressure cooker in that we can only keep the lid on a situation for so long until it blows. It helps clients to appreciate why the teacher is encouraging them to create some space around their difficulties and inviting them to turn towards them with kindness. In this way, difficulties are given some air and the client has a sense of letting off some steam.

"Pain x resistance = Suffering"

This formula enables clients to appreciate the relationship between their difficulties and their experience of suffering. Mindfulness assists in recognising what those difficulties are and seeing that it's their resistance to it, their multifarious defence mechanisms, that result in suffering.

Developing awareness around how the client is resisting their suffering is really what the teacher is exploring through inquiry. The client's unconscious resistance is brought to their consciousness, facilitating their explorations as to how this may impact on their life.

Leaning into the difficulties with kindness can result in developing a level of acceptance, seeing things as they really are and, therefore, reducing suffering. Trying to elicit change is exhausting and huge amounts of energy can be saved by acknowledging that things are just as they are.

Of course, a teacher must keep in mind that resistance can sometimes be helpful in protecting clients from trauma. Rather like a deep-sea diver who must come up slowly from the depths of the ocean to prevent the bends, so too a client may need to take things slowly, giving time to build resources and resilience so that deep-seated difficulties can be explored with kindness, without feeling overwhelmed.

"What we can feel, we can heal"

By not acknowledging difficulties, a client may keep them on lock-down and not be able to work with them by not giving them the air and sunlight necessary to heal. Mindfulness teachers often use the phrase "Mindfulness is not a therapy, but it is therapeutic in nature". What they are referring to is precisely this feeling and healing: opening to the felt sense of experiences so that they can be observed and imbued with compassion.

"If you can name it, you can tame it"

This phrase is particularly useful when identifying mind traps with clients, such as catastrophising and blaming others for their pain. As a result of practice, habitual styles of thinking are recognised. If left unnamed and unchecked, they have the capacity to drive reactive behaviours. However, if a client is able to say to themselves, "This is a catastrophic thought", they are able to go back to a place of observation rather than feelings of being swept away and out of control.

The riverbank analogy is helpful here. I think of thoughts as being akin to a river flowing by whilst one is sitting on the riverbank. One is maintaining a distance from them and simply observing the motion and content. Thinking, or a sense of being overwhelmed by thoughts, feelings, or emotions occurs when standing in the river with everything swishing around, often getting caught up in the current and being washed downstream. This manifests as a feeling of lack of control and submergence, resulting in anxiety and panic.

Naming thoughts has the effect of helping a client to stay on the riverbank!

Prioritising, planning and pacing

It is easy to come across as eager, evangelical even, especially if the teacher is a new one, wishing to impart the joys of mindfulness to others and share their own insights and changes as a result of their own inquiry and discovery process. This, however, can be something of a turn-off for clients, so the teacher may need to rein themselves in from time to time.

Prioritising learning, with the key objectives underpinning the session and returning to them if there's a tendency to aimlessly drift, needs to be balanced with allowing space for things to flow freely. Allowing plenty of time to just "be" within the session, discerning when to deviate and when to maintain boundaries and rigidity, fluctuates within each session and over the course of several sessions.

I often think of mindfulness teaching as a pantomime (a pantomime contains many jokes that children can understand but also includes more subtle ones for the benefit of the adults in the audience). Rather like these different levels of entertainment, a client will only take on board the teaching at the level where they are right now. Some clients are emotionally mature and a teacher can go deeply quite quickly, whereas others may take many sessions to even understand what mindfulness is. It is important to keep the momentum going for everyone in the group and not allow the teaching level to be dictated by the person with the least understanding (it doesn't matter if some aspects of teaching go above their head, they will still be learning at their own level).

It's helpful to plan what the learning for the next session may be – perhaps at the end of a teaching. I always keep notes to remind me of how I'm going to help build clients' understanding of mindfulness through what they've learnt this week. Each session flows from one to the next, building on the learning of the last session, providing scaffolding for growth. This helps to contextualise what has been learnt during a session, giving clients the opportunity to put it into practice in the intervening period, thereby reinforcing learning and connecting with the relational aspects of each session, giving it perspective and deepening understanding of how this learning can be skilfully applied.

Because there appears to be so much learning to get through, and so little time, there is often a tendency to teach too many points, with one falling over the next as the teacher crams as much as possible into each session. By moving on too swiftly from one thing to the next on the agenda there's no room for processing, discussion or reiterating a teaching point. The teacher could ask themselves, "Am I putting so much in to alleviate my own anxieties?"

Through maintaining an awareness of where the teacher is in the course, they can guide the client at the right speed for them. Sometimes it's tempting to try and teach too much as a result of one client's experience. However, if they, or the group as a whole, are not yet ready for that learning, it may not stick. If it's held back, paced well and introduced when appropriate, the client can then contextualise the learning, making it more applicable and accessible.

The length of inquiry is tempered to suit the individual. Some may be reluctant to share at the beginning and this is OK. Just saying, "Thank you", once they've shared an experience is enough to validate and share more later on.

A supervisee was reflecting to me recently that she had feedback from one of her group participants that every comment that anyone made was always related by her back to one of the core features of mindfulness. They said that this felt a little contrived and rigid, which impacted on their desire to share, feeling that it would always be realigned with mindfulness, whatever was said. There is such learning here. We don't always have to have the final say, know the answer, compartmentalise inquiry feedback. Sometimes the best and most skilful thing to do as a teacher is to let the observation just percolate a little, giving it space to land. This is often when true insights happen. When these insights do arise, I may just say something like, "That feels like something very personal just landed. Thank you for sharing it." Then I give it a little space before moving on, without having to dig deeper or explore more fully. This gives the client's emotional mind time to process it without the need for words or cognitions.

Although the teacher may have studied hard, attended numerous workshops, talks, conferences and retreats, and read all the mindfulness books and research available, it is important to remember that the client is their own expert and the teacher's role is to guide and facilitate as much or as little as is necessary for each individual. What the teacher needs to do is gently encourage compassionate exploration of their experiences, asking them to look more closely and investigate more intricately through their own knowledge base. The teacher will never truly know what is there ready to be unearthed but they can provide the safe territory for investigation and discovery.

Indeed, the opposite might be true, and the teacher's role is to enable the participant to pull back a little more, gain some perspective by looking at things from a distance without losing their sense of curiosity. Sometimes we can all become too intimately entwined with our experiences and, as the saying goes, "we can't see the wood for the trees". This really is not helpful sometimes and creating space from a situation, looking at it from a higher viewpoint, can support a participant in finding their bearings once more.

Client/group contract

At the beginning of any session, creating the opportunity to have a conversation about what the client or group needs from this process enables them to feel safe and supported. This group contract may be done quite briefly, setting out some boundaries from the teacher's perspective too, such as the need for confidentiality and for each person to take responsibility for their own needs in each session.

The teacher may wish to explore the issues raised further, to enable each client to be heard and their needs to be validated, something that may be somewhat lacking in their own lives. Some examples may relate to the need to feel respected, valuing individuality, honouring differences, explanations around their behaviour (for example, the need to move every 20 minutes due to a health condition), not wishing to be touched if distressed, requiring kindness and good, clear communication, knowing what is expected of them.

It is helpful to write this on the board in case it needs to be revisited during any of the sessions. It can be used to reground and stabilise the group – a reminder of what was agreed at the outset by each member.

Building the client, teacher and group cohesion via the agreed, self-forming group contract promotes a sense of safety to explore more deeply into the fullness of their experiences. This is often enhanced by tea/coffee, biscuits and cake!

Leading inquiry one-to-one

Much of what I have written about thus far has been more pertinent to working with groups. Over 20 years ago I began this work in a clinical setting, working with clients one-to-one, and I appreciate fully the differences between the two approaches with regards to teaching and inquiry.

When working one-to-one, there's a tendency for the client to reveal more of a personal nature, as inquiry is bespoke to their specific needs and circumstances. There are also no social inhibitory factors, as happens with a group of strangers or colleagues.

The session lengths are usually shorter, one hour being enough to teach practices, contextualise their learning and inquire into their experiences.

Clients suffering with trauma, severe and chronic pain, social anxiety and other presentations often benefit more from this approach, though it might be that one hour is too long. Under these circumstances I would recommend a higher frequency of contact with shortened sessions, perhaps with more support in-between in the form of videos of me leading practices, detailed templates to record experiences and direct conversations via email or telephone.

However, there are also some downsides to working one-to-one. Sometimes more misunderstanding can be apparent in relation to the role of teacher. This often needs clarification, explaining that they're not a therapist, unless of course they are! Explaining that the teacher is a facilitator and doesn't have all the answers deepens a client's understanding of their roles and expectations of each other.

Because of the benefits of joining a group, I may well begin by seeing clients one-to-one and then recommend that they attend a group course, as and when they feel ready to do so. I would explain the difference between the two approaches and spend some time ensuring that the client understands how roles differ in this scenario and that their confidentiality will be maintained. I would not let other group members know that I have been seeing the client one-to-one and would welcome them to the course as if this was the first time we'd met.

The teacher must remain mindful and vigilant that they're not revealing too much about their own personal experiences, as the structure of one-to-one work is looser, often less formal and the relationship can become one of familiarity quite readily. If the teacher reminds themselves of their role and stays in touch with the intentions of the relationship, examples and personal stories will remain pertinent and relevant, for the good of the client.

Maintaining clear notes on what has been said in previous sessions and what it would be helpful to teach next time, as well as the client's potential learning through inquiry, stabilises the process, giving it flow and momentum, in conjunction with balance and equilibrium.

Mindful movement

I have singled this practice out because it is often overlooked by mindfulness teachers who think they don't have the skills or confidence to teach it to others. In my view, being mindful when moving creates a bridge between stillness practices and everyday life, and is one reason why mindfulness has become so accessible. It does not involve going to a quiet place on one's own with specialist equipment but can be integrated with ease into all that we do.

There is profound value in teaching mindful movement, whether in the form of yoga, dance, Pilates, walking, or any form of physical exercise. Paying attention to the body whilst in movement can be a meditative process. Rather than moving mindlessly, rushing from A to B, a client learns to become more attuned to the effects of movement in their body, emotions and thoughts, and can transfer these skills to everyday life. Therefore, if a teacher is able to help their client to acquire this skill in a classroom setting, through the process of inquiry, they create the learning environment to enable them to bring a fresh perspective to their experiences as they go about their day.

For example, in my yoga classes I often ask the group to move into a posture and hold that position, feeling the breath, the muscles starting to work hard, the changing sensations, the mind giving instructions to come out and how they feel emotionally to simply be with that experience. Once they have released the posture, I might inquire as to what their experience was and whether there was some learning in playing with their edge (often their wobble, literally, staying with it without pulling back) and whether there was potential to take this into daily life. Creating a safe environment in which to explore, while being supported by the teacher, facilitates growth and change through accessing other layers of understanding of the self that sitting alone cannot unveil. This resilience training happens in all the realms of experiences, in conjunction with the neurological changes that are stimulated through mindful movement and the connectivity that ensues within a group, especially when all are working just beyond their comfort zone. Compassion is an essential ingredient and enhances the sense that "we're all in this together".

Asking questions such as "What did you do with your discomfort as your legs started to tremble?" or "How did it feel emotionally to hold the position because I [the teacher] was compassionately inviting you to stay there?" can stimulate very helpful, bonding and revolutionary discussions and insights that can become embedded in life beyond the class over time.

Working with established personal and professional relationships

When delivering in a setting where clients already know each other – be it a workplace, friendship group, with clients who are in a relationship of some sort with each other, a social or client group, or elsewhere – a variety of additional considerations need to be taken into account.

An understanding of the pros and cons of working with people who know each other and possibly have a hierarchical relationship is helpful. Although the teacher doesn't need to know all the details from the outset, this knowledge enables them to put boundaries in place and initiate conversations to highlight how this might impact on the clients' learning and processes.

Specifically, in relation to the workplace scenario, these conversations may begin with the organisation that has commissioned the teaching, particularly if the teacher is to deliver a course. In my experience, teaching different levels of staff in the same group means that they are unable to be open about their full experiences. It is preferable to offer teaching where participants are generally at the same staffing level, where they have more freedom to explore specific issues at work without feeling too guarded. These discussions will also shape the use of assessment tools before and after teaching and the intentions of the organisation for inviting the teacher to deliver sessions. Inquiry can then be more focused on these issues, such as building resilience, helping staff manage transitions or creating cultural change from within.

The teacher would address this situation openly with each client, individually, during the assessment process, asking questions around how they feel being taught alongside their colleagues, whether they have any difficulties with anyone that they think the teacher should be informed about, how they're feeling about work at the moment and any other issues that might arise.

Considerations and information relating to their personal data, confidentiality, how the teacher and organisation will gather, store, analyse, utilise and dispose of personal details before, during and after the course is important. A piece of written information detailing these aspects and a signature showing consent may be required.

The teacher should consider exactly what they are being asked to deliver and give advice on the minimum and maximum number of attendees in any cohort. This depends on a range of factors, including expectations, teaching content, longevity of delivery, experience of the teacher, availability and engagement of staff, facilities and timings available and the context of teaching. All these factors will impact on the inquiry process too (for example, in the form of group collusion, in-jokes or undercurrents around discussion topics that the teacher is unaware of).

A positive aspect of teaching those who know each other is the support they are able to share. Going through the process together is a very bonding experience. They can develop systems such as meditation buddies or set up their own meditation practice group through a shared platform, practice together at work and even create a room specifically for mindfulness practice. They are also able to be creative in how they introduce a mindful attitude into their work and continue with their learning and development, way beyond the end of the programme.

Teamwork

Mindfulness has the capacity to contribute to creating the environment for the development of high-performing teams. Having introduced and delivered a Mindful Leadership programme for Somerset Council's social work team leaders over the last five years,[5] I found that outcomes revealed higher levels of engagement, connectivity, self-efficacy, emotional regulation and self-compassion.

Teams can benefit from the sense that they're learning together to communicate more effectively, listening more deeply to the ideas and needs of their colleagues, and introducing, in practical ways, what they have learnt into their meetings, their working relationships, supervision and all aspects of work within the team.

This leads to an inner feeling of safety, value and security which manifests as being more creative, open, healthier and happier at work.

The use of tools

Tools can be used to great effect to stimulate inquiry, helping clients to put into context what they are experiencing via visual aids, pen and paper exercises and other creative teaching strategies.

Inquiry comes in all manner of ways and the teacher will have their own toolbox of quotes, objects, diagrams, stories and poetry to hand, as these different resources can be powerful tools, engaging interest and learning. Sometimes I leave the message of the poem or story to filter in, perhaps pausing after the reading. However, I do

---

5   MindfulnessUK and Somerset County Council (2015–2019) Mindful Leadership Programme for Social Work Team Leaders.

think that it can also be a helpful device to inquire into the effects of the reading. These resources often create a sense of connecting and "landing" and so provide the opportunity and fertile ground for deepening into inquiry.

I incorporate a range of these tools within any teaching context, giving the client something to work with and develop a deeper appreciation of what they are experiencing during practice and how this can relate, in a practical way, to their everyday life experiences.

These tools would have been explored during any mindfulness teacher training and will be very familiar to anyone teaching mindfulness. Importantly, whatever is used must be client-centred and the teacher should have a clear intention for teaching them, so that inquiry can be guided in an applied way.

Journaling can be one of these tools, the teacher providing a template to use, such as the practice and self-inquiry diary given in the Appendix. I encourage clients to journal: to commit their experiences to paper, audio or in some other format. This serves multifarious functions and I see it as a positive support to the process of inquiry. It is fair to say that some clients relish this process and others are less engaged, but there is ample room for creativity here. My personal preference is to use audio to record my experiences after practice, or the effects of mindfulness on my life, as it takes less time and feels more experiential as a process. A great book, *A Philosophy of Walking* (Gros 2015), explores the wonderful ways in which thoughts have led to great pieces of philosophical work and revelations over the centuries, whilst walking with these thoughts being scribed to ensure they were accurately recorded in the moment.

Offering support, encouragement, advice, and templates on which to record experiences after practice, can then be inquired upon during the next teaching session. Sometimes I might ask a client to bring in their journal to discuss their reflections as this can have a profound effect on the client's engagement with inquiry and assists the development of their self-inquiry skills.

Finding and developing a compassionate mindful community

My compassionate mindful community is one of the most important aspects of my life. Being authentically supported by others who are also inquiring into their own experiences and exploring meditation to deepen into their understanding of themselves and others, with kindness, makes my heart sing and gives me such strength and courage.

It's no real surprise, therefore, that I have incorporated the development of a community into my life's work, both personally and professionally, widening the borders of my community with every passing year.

Clients who are just starting to learn about mindfulness are placing their foot on the first rung of a ladder. Support in the form of considering "what's next" for the client is of profound importance for some. The teacher can play a significant role in helping clients to continue on this path, depending on what they request or need. There is such a range of ways to provide this ongoing support and facilitation of inquiry through sitting groups, online teaching, signposting to like-minded organisations, reading lists, retreats, refresher courses, establishing connections through social media, meditation platforms, podcasts, apps and an abundance of other creative ways.

Once one starts to become aware that mindfulness might be the key to developing a new way of living a rich, fulfilling and more compassionate life, regular practice has the potential to reap boundless and unending rewards.

Stephanie Unthank[6] explains how things have changed for her, as a result of practising mindfulness and subsequently training to teach mindfulness and compassion to others:

It's about moral compass for me, what do I stand for? What's within my gift to offer society?

My values and integrity guide me in my day-to-day decision-making, I know when something feels right.

Paying it forward always brings rewards, monetary or otherwise, but the biggest personal reward in my working with others is experience, opportunity, meeting new people, helping to put smiles on people's faces, simply just helping others in any way I can, is what motivates me.

Since I came to mindfulness and left the corporate world behind, the simple attitude of non-striving has brought me so much peace (and success).

---

6   Personal communication (2019) with Stephanie Unthank (wellness professional).

In the world we live in, we will always have these challenges, so we face into them, do what's right, and live by our own moral codes and values.

Practising mindfulness is just the start. Go deeper and the fruits of practice have the potential to enrich the lives of every single one of us, creating a world of compassionate mindful connection in which all living beings can thrive and flourish.

Appendix

Frequently asked questions (FAQs)

Clients often ask similar questions, relating to both formal and informal practices. These FAQs are given to help the teacher think about how they might answer these inquiry questions, in advance.

Shorter practices

- How often do I have to do these practices?

- How long do they take as I don't have much time?

- Do I have to get into a meditative posture, away from my work and family?

- If I just do these, will that be enough to make the brain changes I've heard so much about?

- I just can't remember to do them, what do you suggest I can do to remind myself?

Longer practices
Body scan

- How do I stop myself falling asleep?

- What am I looking for during the practice?

- My thoughts go out in all directions and I feel like I'm wrestling with them. How can I stop this happening and focus on the practice?

- It's difficult to find the time – I'm always on alert at home. When is the best time to practice?

- I start to itch, which is distracting. Should I scratch or resist?

- I get really bored. What does that mean?

- I want it to be just right and it's irritating when it's not. How can I make it right?

- I feel agitated before the practice, as I have to squeeze it into my day. Should I do something beforehand so I can settle better?

Mindful movement practice

- I preferred the body scan. Can I go back to that?

- I now anticipate what is coming next, so my mind is wandering more, the more I do it.

- I feel resistant to it as I want perfection. Is this usual?

- What do I do if I feel soreness or pain?

- Can I change some of the exercises if I can't do the ones on the recording?

Breathing practice

- Do I need to deepen my breathing?

- Am I allowed to move if I feel uncomfortable?

- I feel anxious when I focus on my breath. What can I do?

- Can I do this any time I like?

- What should I do if I can't feel any movement in my abdomen?

Coping strategies

- How often do I have to do these?

- Should I practice them only when I feel stressed?

- Should I take really deep breaths in when I'm feeling panicky?

Daily activities

- The activities are making me more stressed as I feel like they're making me dawdle, when I have so much to do. Can I speed back up to normal pace?

- I can only do it with my eyes closed. Is this OK?

- I love getting completely absorbed in knitting/drawing. Is this mindfulness?

- Do I have to do every activity mindfully, because I don't understand how I can make plans if I'm constantly in the moment?

SHORT EMAILED CLIENT ASSESSMENT FORM

Thank you for filling out this form. We realise the personal nature of these questions and please be assured that they are kept in strict confidence adhering to the General Data Protection Regulation (GDPR), 2018. The data will be kept for the duration of the course. On completion of the course you may request that the information be returned to you or disposed of from our records.

Name: . . . .

Contact email: . . . .

Telephone: . . . .

Course dates you are intending to attend: . . . .

Course venue: . . . .

Date this form is completed: . . . .

Questions

- Do you know anything about mindfulness? Please give details.

  . . . .

  . . . .

  . . . .

  . . . .

  . . . .

- What is your main reason for wishing to participate in this course?

  . . . .

  . . . .

  . . . .

  . . . .

  . . . .

- Although this is not a therapy group, it is helpful to know if there are any significant personal issues going on in your life. Please provide details. (This can be discussed in confidence when the more detailed assessment is being taken, in person.)

  . . . .

  . . . .

  . . . .

  . . . .

  . . . .

- Between sessions there is an expectation that you do guided home practices for a minimum of 30 minutes per day, plus additional short exercises and strategies.

  Do you have time to do this? Please circle   Yes/No

  When and where would that be? . . . .

- Do you have any difficulties that I need to know about so that I can support your learning? Please give details if applicable.

  Pain . . . .

  Mobility . . . .

  Props to make you more comfortable . . . .

  Supportive chair required . . . .

  Hard of hearing . . . .

  Interpreter required . . . .

  Other . . . .

Information for you

Here are details of the venue and parking.

Please wear comfortable clothing. There are changing facilities if required.

. . . .

. . . .

. . . .

Do you have any further questions about the practicalities around the course?

. . . .

. . . .

. . . .

. . . .

. . . .

. . . .

Do you have any questions of any sort or is there anything else we can help you with to support your attendance on the course?

. . . .

. . . .

. . . .

. . . .

. . . .

. . . .

Please complete the form and return it to xxxxxxxx. The teacher will then contact you directly, prior to course commencement, and go through a more detailed assessment with you. This also gives you the opportunity to discuss any questions or issues arising for you, in confidence.

FULL CLIENT ASSESSMENT FORM

NAME:		Date:		
ADDRESS:				
TELEPHONE:	Day:	Eve:		Mobile:
EMAIL:		DOB:		
OCCUPATION:				
Doctor's details if applicable:				
How did you find out about MindfulnessUK? Referral or self-referral?				
Main reason for attending?				
What are your intention and expectations of mindfulness and the teacher?				
Please identify three goals	....			
Have you been hospitalised in the last year for any reason? Please give details				
Are you on any prescribed medication? Do you take any recreational drugs? Please give details				

Do you have any physical, psychological, emotional, lifestyle or attitudinal issues? [Suicidality, if appropriate]	
Have you suffered with any trauma or significant difficulties that would be helpful for the teacher to know about? Please give details	

Do you suffer from any of the following conditions?:

Anxiety	Cancer	Disc problems	Hearing difficulties
Arthritis	Suicidal thoughts	Depression	
Panic attacks	IBS	Headaches, dizziness, epilepsy, vertigo or difficulties concentrating	Digestive complaints
High or low blood pressure	Back, neck or knee pain		Menstrual or hormonal problems
Asthma or other breathing problems	Diabetes		
	Glaucoma or eye problems	Heart or circulation problems	Broken, fractured or dislocated bones in past two years
Artificial joints			

Sleep patterns	
Allergies/ sensitivities	
Treatments from other health professionals in the last three years	
Support at work, home and socially	

Practical considerations	
How many sessions can you commit to? How much time do you have to do home practice? Do you have any questions regarding the practice?	
Do you have any difficulties that we need to know about so I can support your learning (e.g. hard of hearing, padded chair, interpreter, CD, printed handouts)?	

Lifestyle questions			
Smoke	............./day	Diet	
Drink: tea	............./day		
Drink: coffee	............./day		
Drink: alcohol	............./day	Exercise	
Drink: other fluids	............./day		
Hobbies/ relaxation			
Stress levels			

Past meditation/mindfulness experience	
What?	
Where?	
How long?	
Response and support?	

Past yoga or other mindful movement practice			
Type?			
When?			
Response?			
Please complete the next section if you experience pain			
When is pain worst?	Morning Afternoon Evening Night		
How much does pain interfere with sleep?			
Does not interfere 0 1 2 3 4 5 6 7 8 9 10 Completely interferes			
Name three things that make the pain better and three that make it worse			
Better			
Worse			
Is there anything else we can do for you to support your learning?			

Consent

Everything you share with me is strictly confidential and will only be shared with another professional if you or someone else is at risk.

All information is stored and destroyed in adherence with the General Data Protection Regulation (GDPR), 2018.

All the information I (client) have provided is true on the date given.

Date: ....

Signed by client: ....

Signed by teacher: ....

One-Week Practice and Self-Inquiry Diary

Date and time of practice	Practice: Short Long Coping Daily activity	Duration	What did you notice?	How does this help?	What do you need to do now or next?

Glossary

Acetylcholine: Neurotransmitter involved in learning, memory, arousal, attention and inhibition.

Amygdalae: Almond-shaped structures in the brain that detect fear and process emotion.

Anterior: Anatomical term relating to the front part of a structure or region.

Cognitive processes: Processes involved in decision-making, planning and analysing.

Dopamine: Neurotransmitter involved in motivation, reward and pleasure.

Dorsal: Anatomical term relating to the upper part of a structure or region.

GABA: Neurotransmitter involved in inhibition and the reduction of anxiety.

Glutamate: Neurotransmitter involved in facilitation, learning and memory.

Hippocampus: Structure of the brain that is involved in learning and memory.

Lateral: Anatomical term relating to the side part of a structure or region.

Medial: Anatomical term relating to the medium part of a structure or region.

Mirror neurons: Types of neurons in the brain that fire when an animal acts and when they see that same action in another animal, thereby mirroring the behaviour of others.

Posterior: Anatomical term relating to the back part of a structure or region.

Prefrontal cortex: Frontal region of the brain involved in decision-making and memory.

Serotonin: Neurotransmitter involved in perception, mood, sleep and appetite.

Ventral: Anatomical term relating to the lower part of a structure or region.

References

Alexander, B.K., Hadaway, P. & Coambs, R. (1980) 'Rat park chronicle.' *British Columbia Medical Journal* 22(2), 32–45.

Bowen, S., Chawla, N. & Martlatt, G.A. (2010) *Mindfulness-Based Relapse Prevention for Addictive Behaviors: A Clinician's Guide.* New York, NY: Guilford Press.

British Association of Mindfulness-Based Approaches (2019) *Good Practice Guidelines for Mindfulness Teachers.* Available at www.bamba.org.uk.

Collins English Dictionary (2019) 'Inquiry.' Accessed on 04/10/2018 at www.collinsdictionary.com/dictionary/english/inquiry 1.

Donne, J. (1959) *Devotions upon Emergent Occasions.* Ann Arbor, MI: University of Michigan Press. Originally published in London in 1624.

Gilbert, P. (2009) *The Compassionate Mind.* London: Constable and Robinson.

Gros, F. (2015) *A Philosophy of Walking.* London: Verso.

Hanh, T.N. (2001) *Anger: Buddhist Wisdom for Cooling the Flames.* New York, NY: Riverhead Books.

Heads, G. (2017) *Living Mindfully: Discovering Authenticity through Mindfulness Coaching.* Chichester: John Wiley and Sons.

Hölzel, B.K., Carmody, J., Vangel, M., Congleton, C. *et al.* (2011) 'Mindfulness practice leads to increases in regional brain gray matter density.' *Psychiatry Research: Neuroimaging* 191(1), 36–43.

Jarrett, C. (2014) *Great Myths of the Brain.* Hoboken, NJ: John Wiley and Sons.

Kabat-Zinn, J. (2013) *Full Catastrophe Living.* London: Piatkus.

Kabat-Zinn, J. & Santorelli, S. (1999) *Mindfulness-Based Stress Reduction Professional Training Resource Manual.* Worcester, MA: University of Massachusetts Medical School, Center for Mindfulness in Medicine, Health Care, and Society.

Lazar, S.W., Kerr, C.E., Wasserman, R.H., Gray, J.R. *et al.* (2005) 'Meditation experience is associated with increased cortical thickness.' *Neuroreport* 16(17), 1893–1897.

Lomas, T., Edginton, T., Cartwright, T. & Ridge, D. (2014) 'Men developing emotional intelligence through meditation? Integrating narrative, cognitive and electroencephalography (EEG) evidence.' *Psychology of Men & Masculinity, 15*(2), 213–224.

Lutz, A., Slagter, H.A., Dunne, J.D. & Davidson, R.J. (2008) 'Attention regulation and monitoring in meditation.' *Trends in Cognitive Science* 12(4), 163–169.

Lyubomirsky, S. (2010) *The How of Happiness: A Practical Guide to Getting the Life You Want.* London: Piatkus.

Maguire, E.A., Gadian, D.G., Johnsrude, I.S., Good, C.D. *et al.* (2000) 'Navigation-related structural change in the hippocampi of taxi drivers.' *Proceedings of the National Academy of Sciences 97*(8), 4398–4403.

McCown, D, Micozzi, M. & Reibel, D.K. (2011) *Teaching Mindfulness: A Practical Guide for Clinicians and Educators.* New York, NY: Springer.

McTaggart, L. (2003) *The Field.* Glasgow: HarperCollins Publishers.

Norman, D.A. & Shallice, T. (1980) 'Attention to Action: Willed and Automatic Control of Behavior.' In R.J. Davidson, G.E. Schwartz & D. Shapiro (eds) *Consciousness and Self-Regulation.* New York, NY: Plenum.

Rosenberg, M.B. (2003) *Nonviolent Communication* (2nd edn). Encinitas, CA: Puddle Dancer Press.

Tuckman, B. (1965) 'Developmental sequence in small groups.' *Psychological Bulletin 63*, 384–399.

Subject Index

Author Index

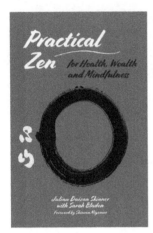

Practical Zen for Health, Wealth and Mindfulness
Julian Daizan Skinner with Sarah Bladen

Paperback: £9.99 / $16.95
ISBN: 978 1 84819 390 1
eISBN: 978 0 85701 347 7

192 pages

Bringing the body-mind insights of Rinzai Zen from the mountains of Japan to the Western world, Zen master Julian Daizan Skinner and Sarah Bladen present simple meditation techniques to help achieve health, wellbeing and success.

Taking the reader through the first 100 days of practice, the book then shows how to adapt the new learned techniques to the rest of your life.

Including case studies at the end of each chapter to show how people's lives have been transformed through their meditation journeys, this is an accessible and practical guide to adapting Eastern meditation into busy Western lives.

Beginning full-time monastic Zen in 1989, **Julian Daizan Skinner** has practiced and received Dharma transmission in the Soto and Rinzai traditions and been named successor of Zen Master Miyamae Shinzan, founder of The Zendo Kyodan Lineage. For more information, visit zenways.org. **Sarah Bladen** is a journalist and Zen meditation teacher active primarily in London and the Middle East.

The Compassionate Practitioner

How to Create a Successful and Rewarding Practice

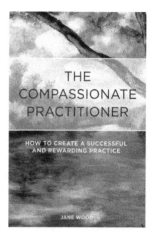

Jane Wood

Paperback: £15.99 / $24.95
ISBN: 978 1 84819 222 5
eISBN: 978 0 85701 170 1

208 pages

Focusing on the importance of relationship-building, this handbook explains how to turn new clients into regulars and make your practice flourish.

If you can create trust, loyalty and a sense of safety in new clients, they are more likely to commit to the further appointments needed to experience the healing you have to offer. This book considers how best to enhance the client's experience at every stage of the consultation through compassion and mindfulness. It is full of practical advice about everything from creating the right ambience in the therapy room to maintaining a positive attitude through self-reflection.

This will be a valued support for students and professionals working in a wide range of complementary and alternative therapies, as well as art, music and drama therapists.

Jane Wood is a teacher, supervisor, workshop facilitator and retired homeopathic practitioner. She is a supervisor and teacher of reflective practice at the University of Westminster and is the head of practitioner development and reflective practice at the International School of Homeopathy, London. She lives in London, UK.

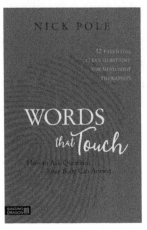

Words that Touch

How to Ask Questions Your Body Can Answer – 12 Essential 'Clean Questions' for Mind/Body Therapists

Nick Pole

Paperback: £18.99 / $27.95
ISBN: 978 1 84819 336 9
eISBN: 978 0 85701 292 0

352 pages

In this practical guide, Nick Pole explains the philosophy and practice of Clean Language, a simple and highly effective way to facilitate mind/body communication in bodywork therapy. He explains how to use language to get to the heart of a client's physical problem, to engage the mind in the process of the body, and to create somatic change.

Words that Touch provides compelling theoretical explanations and practical case studies to describe the importance of language and relationships in the practice of mind/body therapies. Practitioners of yoga, shiatsu, acupuncture, physiotherapy, The Feldenkrais Technique and more will find the guide transformative in increasing the connection with clients and developing their practice through language.

Nick Pole has been a mind-body therapist for over 25 years, and discovered Clean Language after training in shiatsu and NLP. Nick is based in London.

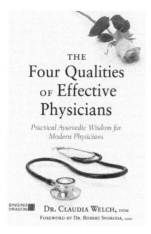

THE
Four Qualities
of Effective
Physicians

Practical Ayurvedic Wisdom for Modern Physicians

Dr. Claudia Welch, dom

Foreword by Dr. Robert Svoboda, mapa

The Four Qualities of Effective Physicians

Practical Ayurvedic Wisdom for Modern Physicians

Dr. Claudia Welch, DOM

Foreword by Dr. Robert Svoboda

Paperback: £12.99 / $17.95
ISBN: 978 1 84819 339 0
eISBN: 978 0 85701 181 7

256 pages

What defines an excellent doctor? He or she must certainly have a wealth of scientific knowledge and practical experience – but is that enough?

Dr Claudia Welch explores how the effectiveness of a physician extends far beyond the ability to prescribe correct treatments, identifying how to enhance the efficacy of medicine using four core doctoring principals: theoretical knowledge, practical experience, dexterity and 'purity'.

Drawing on ancient Eastern medical traditions, modern Western science and her own experience, Dr Welch examines how we know what we know, the mechanics of doctor-patient emotional contagion, and the degree to which a patient's sensory experience in a medical office affects their experience of treatments delivered. She also offers practical steps to cultivating more refined perceptive abilities and improving results.

Dr Welch's book will be essential reading for all healthcare practitioners interested in understanding how to enhance the therapeutic outcomes of their practice, including doctors of Ayurveda, Chinese medicine and Naturopathy, as well as Western medical professionals and other complementary health practitioners.

Claudia Welch is a Doctor of Oriental Medicine, an Ayurvedic practitioner and educator, and the author of Balance Your Hormones, Balance Your Life: Achieving Optimal Health and Wellness Through Ayurveda, Chinese Medicine and Western Science. Dr. Welch lectures internationally on Oriental and Ayurvedic medicines and Women's Health, bringing a depth of knowledge and a sense of joy to her presentations that has established her as a leading educator in the field of Ayurveda. She has served on the teaching faculty of The Ayurvedic Institute, Kripalu School of Ayurveda, Southwest Acupuncture College, and Acupractice Seminars.

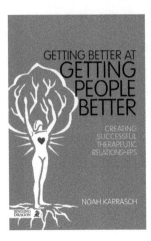

Getting Better at Getting People Better
Creating Successful Therapeutic Relationships
Noel Karrasch

Paperback: £17.99 / $28.95
ISBN: 978 1 84819 239 3
eISBN: 978 0 85701 186 2

192 pages

What is it that really gets people better? With practical information on how to support clients' healing processes, this book helps practitioners across a wide range of physical and medical therapies, as well as psychotherapists, to improve their practice and get better at what they do.

Getting to the core of true healing, Noah Karrasch explores the essentials of effective practice that apply across all healing modalities and expands on a four step formula based on these essentials: caring about patrons, providing a safe setting, communicating with clients, and encouraging their participation in their own healing. The book also discusses the practitioner's self-understanding and self-healing work as a vital part of becoming a better provider of health and healing, and Karrasch presents a model of communication focused on recognising which of four centers (head, heart, gut, or groin) both practitioners and their clients operate from to strengthen ties between healing partners.

Revealing the fundamentals of effective practice drawn from a wide range of therapies, this book provides practical advice, as well as points of reflection, for all those seeking to deepen their therapeutic practice.

Noah Karrasch is a licensed deep tissue massage therapist and holds a teaching degree from the University of Missouri, Columbia. He teaches CORE bodywork skills around the world. He lives and works in Springfield, Missouri.

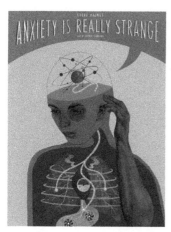

Anxiety is Really Strange
Steve Haines
Art by Sophie Standing

Paperback: £7.99 / $12.95
ISBN: 978 1 84819 389 5
Hardback: £12.99 / $17.99
ISBN: 978 1 84819 407 6
eISBN: 978 0 85701 345 3

32 pages

Highly Commended in the 2018 British Medical Association Book Awards.

What is the difference between fear and excitement and how can you tell them apart? How do the mind and body make emotions? When can anxiety be good? This science-based graphic book addresses these questions and more, revealing just how strange anxiety is, but also how to unravel its mysteries and relieve its effects.

Understanding how anxiety is created by our nervous system trying to protect us, and how our fight-or-flight mechanisms can get stuck, can significantly lessen the fear experienced during anxiety attacks. In this guide, anxiety is explained in an easy-to-understand, engaging graphic format with tips and strategies to relieve its symptoms, and change the mind's habits for a more positive outlook.

Steve Haines has studied Yoga, Shiatsu, Biodynamic Craniosacral Therapy, and Trauma Releasing Exercises and works in healthcare and as a UK registered Chiropractor. Steve is the bestselling author of *Pain is Really Strange* and *Trauma is Really Strange*. He lives between London and Geneva. (www.stevehaines.net).

Sophie Standing is a London-based illustrator and designer, specialising in human sciences. Her style combines digital and hand-made, with an emphasis on rich colour, textures and metaphorical concepts.

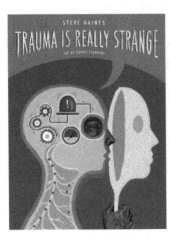

Trauma is Really Strange
Steve Haines
Art by Sophie Standing

Paperback: £7.99 / $12.95
ISBN: 978 1 84819 293 5
eISBN: 978 0 85701 240 1

32 pages

What is trauma? How does it change the way our brains work? And how can we overcome it?

When something traumatic happens to us, we dissociate and our bodies shut down their normal processes. This unique comic explains the strange nature of trauma and how it confuses the brain and affects the body. With wonderful artwork, cat and mouse metaphors, essential scientific facts, and a healthy dose of wit, the narrator reveals how trauma resolution involves changing the body's physiology and describes techniques that can achieve this, including Trauma Releasing Exercises that allow the body to shake away tension, safely releasing deep muscular patterns of stress and trauma.

Steve Haines has studied Yoga, Shiatsu, Biodynamic Craniosacral Therapy, and Trauma Releasing Exercises and works in healthcare and as a UK registered Chiropractor. Steve is the bestselling author of *Pain is Really Strange* and *Trauma is Really Strange*. He lives between London and Geneva. (www.stevehaines.net).

Sophie Standing is a London-based illustrator and designer, specialising in human sciences. Her style combines digital and hand-made, with an emphasis on rich colour, textures and metaphorical concepts.

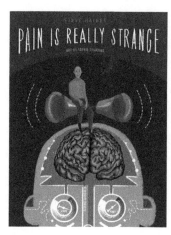

Pain is Really Strange

Steve Haines

Art by Sophie Standing

Paperback: £7.99 / $12.95
ISBN: 978 1 84819 264 5
Hardback: £12.99 / $17.99
ISBN: 978 1 84819 366 6
eISBN: 978 0 85701 212 8

32 pages

Answering questions such as 'how can I change my pain experience?', 'what is pain?', and 'how do nerves work?', this short research-based graphic book reveals just how strange pain is and explains how understanding it is often the key to relieving its effects.

Studies show that understanding how pain is created and maintained by the nervous system can significantly lessen the pain you experience. The narrator in this original, gently humorous book explains pain in an easy-to-understand, engaging graphic format and reveals how to change the mind's habits to transform pain.

Steve Haines has studied Yoga, Shiatsu, Biodynamic Craniosacral Therapy, and Trauma Releasing Exercises and works in healthcare and as a UK registered Chiropractor. Steve is the bestselling author of *Pain is Really Strange* and *Trauma is Really Strange*. He lives between London and Geneva. (www.stevehaines.net).

Sophie Standing is a London-based illustrator and designer, specialising in human sciences. Her style combines digital and hand-made, with an emphasis on rich colour, textures and metaphorical concepts.

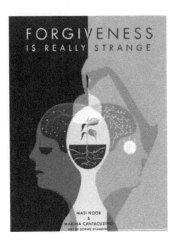

Forgiveness is Really Strange

Masi Noor and Maria Cantacuzino

Art by Sophie Standing

Hardback: £9.99 / $14.95
ISBN: 978 1 78592 124 7
eISBN: 978 0 85701 279 1

64 pages

What is forgiveness? What enables people to forgive? Why do we even choose to forgive those who have harmed us? What can the latest psychological research tell us about the nature of forgiveness, its benefits and risks?

This imaginative comic explores the key aspects of forgiveness, asking what it means to forgive and to be forgiven. Witty and intelligent, it answers questions about the health benefits and restorative potential of forgiveness and explains, in easy-to-understand terms, what happens in our brains, bodies and communities when we choose to forgive.

Dr Masi Noor is a Senior Lecturer in Social Psychology at the University of Keele with a special interest in forgiveness as a possible conflict resolution strategy. Together with Marina Cantacuzino, he created The Forgiveness Toolbox (www.theforgivenesstoolbox.com). Masi is based in Keele, UK.

Marina Cantacuzino is an award-winning journalist and founder of The Forgiveness Project (www.theforgivenessproject.com), a charitable organisation that uses real personal narratives to explore how ideas around forgiveness, reconciliation and conflict resolution can be used to impact positively on people's lives. She is based in London, UK.

Sophie Standing is a London-based illustrator and designer, specialising in human sciences. Her style combines digital and hand-made, with an emphasis on rich colour, textures and metaphorical concepts. She is also the illustrator of *Pain is Really Strange* and *Trauma is Really Strange.* www.sophiestandingillustration.com